Die Infektion beim Brandverletzten

Stephan Lorenz, Peter-Rudolf Zellner (Hrsg.)

Die Infektion beim Brandverletzten

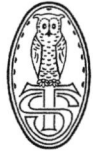 Steinkopff Verlag Darmstadt

Anschrift der Herausgeber:
Stephan Lorenz
Kreiskrankenhaus Lüdenscheid
Chirurgie I
Paulmannshöher Straße 14
58516 Lüdenscheid

Prof. Dr. Dr. med. Peter-Rudolf Zellner
Atos Praxisklinik Heidelberg
Bismarckstraße 9–15
69115 Heidelberg

Die Deutsche Bibliothek – CIP-Einheitsaufnahme

Die Infektion beim Brandverletzten / Stefan Lorenz ; Peter-Rudolf Zellner (Hrsg.). – Darmstadt : Steinkopff, 1993

ISBN-13:978-3-642-85420-0   e-ISBN-13:978-3-642-85419-4
DOI: 10.1007/978-3-642-85419-4

NE: Lorenz, Stephan [Hrsg.]

Dieses Werk ist urheberrechtlich geschützt. Die dadurch begründeten Rechte, insbesondere die der Übersetzung, des Nachdrucks, des Vortrages, der Entnahme von Abbildungen und Tabellen, der Funksendung, der Mikroverfilmung oder der Vervielfältigung auf anderen Wegen und der Speicherung in Datenverarbeitungsanlagen, bleiben, auch bei nur auszugsweiser Verwertung, vorbehalten. Eine Vervielfältigung dieses Werkes oder von Teilen dieses Werkes ist auch im Einzelfall nur in den Grenzen der gesetzlichen Bestimmungen des Urheberrechtsgesetzes der Bundesrepublik Deutschland vom 9. September 1965 in der Fassung vom 24. Juni 1985 zulässig. Sie ist grundsätzlich vergütungspflichtig. Zuwiderhandlungen unterliegen den Strafbestimmungen des Urheberrechtsgesetzes.

Copyright © 1993 by Dr. Dietrich Steinkopff Verlag, GmbH & Co. KG Darmstadt
Softcover reprint of the hardcover 1st edition 1993
Verlagsredaktion: Jens Fabry – English Editor: James C. Willis – Herstellung: Heinz J. Schäfer

Die Wiedergabe von Gebrauchsnamen, Handelsnamen, Warenbezeichnungen usw. in dieser Veröffentlichung berechtigt auch ohne besondere Kennzeichnung nicht zu der Annahme, daß solche Namen im Sinne der Warenzeichen- und Markenschutz-Gesetzgebung als frei zu betrachten wären und daher von jedermann benutzt werden dürften.

Gesamtherstellung: Konrad Triltsch, Würzburg
Gedruckt auf säurefreiem Papier

Vorwort

Die Infektion stellt nach wie vor ein kardinales Problem bei der Behandlung brandverletzter Patienten dar. Fortschritte auf dem Gebiet der Plastischen Chirurgie und der Intensivmedizin haben zwar geholfen, die Prognose bei schweren Verbrennungen wesentlich zu verbessern, bergen aber auch neue Gefahren, die sich auch und im besonderen als infektiöse Komplikationen manifestieren. Erkenntnisse über die Pathophysiologie des Verbrennungstraumas und der Sepsis weisen neue Therapieansätze auf und stellen konventionelle Behandlungsschemata teilweise in Frage. Die Bewährungsprobe im klinischen Alltag steht jedoch zum größten Teil noch aus.

Im März 1992 fand deshalb zu dem Thema „Die Infektion beim Brandverletzten" ein Symposium in Ludwigshafen statt. In einer Zusammenschau wurden aktuelle Erkenntnisse über Pathologie und Pathophysiologie septischer Komplikationen, Ätiologie der Infektion, Infektionswege und Infektionskontrolle beim Brandverletzten beleuchtet. Verbrennungsmediziner aus dem In- und Ausland referierten und diskutierten ihre Therapiekonzepte. In diesem Buch sind die wichtigsten Beiträge des Symposiums zusammengefaßt. Es wendet sich an alle, die direkt oder indirekt mit der Behandlung von Verbrennungen befaßt sind, soll aber insbesondere dem Kliniker Denkanstöße und Hilfestellung bei der täglichen Arbeit bieten.

Lüdenscheid, Juni 1993   Die Herausgeber

Inhaltsverzeichnis

Vorwort V

The history of burn care in the U.S.A.
J. Boswick 1

Pathologie und Pathophysiologie des Verbrennungstraumas

Cause of mortality in thermally injured patients
W. G. Cioffi, S. H. Kim, and B. A. Pruitt, Jr. 7

Pathologie und Pathophysiologie des Verbrennungstraumas
K. Wegener 13

Pathogenetische Mechanismen der verbrennungsinduzierten Immunsuppression
M. Köller, J. Brom und W. König 25

The hypermetabolism of major thermal burn: Implications for infections
D. N. Herndon, T. C. Rutan, and D. Fleming 37

Ätiologie der Infektion, Infektionswege, Infektionskontrolle

Analyse des Keimspektrums und der Übertragungswege auf einer Verbrennungsintensivstation
D. Kistler, R. Jurek und R. Hettich 45

Use of burn wound biopsies in the diagnosis and treatment of burn wound infection
B. A. Pruitt, Jr., A. T. MacManus, S. H. Kim, and W. G. Cioffi 55

The problem of lung infection in extensive burns
J. Gilbaud and Y. Legulluche 65

Die Beatmungstherapie beim Brandverletzten – Komplikationen und Outcome
R. Stuttmann 79

Microbial translocation following burn injury
J. W. Alexander and L. Gianotti 95

Therapie

Topical and surgical treatment of the burn wound
D. N. Herndon, R. L. Rutan, and T. C. Rutan 107

Die konservative und operative Therapie der Brandwunde
P. R. Zellner, T. Raff und S. Lorenz 113

Hyperbaric oxygen therapy in the treatment of thermal burns
P. E. Cianci 123

Die Antibiotikatherapie beim Brandverletzten
G. Germann 135

Human monoclonal antibodies for therapy of *Pseudomonas* infections
D. Rohm 149

Measurement of sepsis in the burn patient
A. M. Munster, M. Smith-Meek, D. Zhou, C. Dickerson,
and R. A. Winchurch 153

Die Therapie der Sepsis
G. Germann 161

The history of burn care in the U.S.A.

J. Boswick

Denver, U.S.A.

I was pleased to be asked to speak on the history of burn care in the USA, because this provided an opportunity to review certain aspects of burn care, the development of burn care facilities, and the contribution of many individuals to the progress of burn care in the USA during the past five to six decades.

It is not possible in the time allocated to review all the important developments of burn care, to recognize all the individuals who made significant contributions, or to mention all of the institutions where burn care has been significantly advanced during this time. Therefore, I will direct my remarks to certain events, individuals and institutions that I have known personally.

Some of the most historic and important developments are in the field of fluid resuscitation for the prevention and occasional treatment of burn shock.

One of the early events that is often credited with stimulating an interest in fluid resuscitation for burn patients was the work of Dr. Francis Moore of Boston, who had the opportunity of studying a large group of patients who sustained burn injuries from a night club fire often referred to as the Cocoanut Grove disaster. Dr. Moore's work stimulated many others to become interested in fluid replacement for burn and other trauma patients.

Dr. Everett Evans of Richmond, Virginia, became interested in this problem and developed a formula for planning fluid replacement in burn patients. The staff at Brooke Army Medical Center unit was also interested in fluid resuscitation for burn patients and proposed a slightly different formula for this purpose. In addition, Drs. Carl Moyer, Thomas Shires, and Charles Baxter at Parkland Hospital in Dallas studied fluid problems in burn and trauma patients and developed a formula for burn and trauma patients that utilized only a balanced salt solution for early resuscitation within the first 48 hours. Others working in this field have made other recommendations which I will mention later.

Another important recent event in the history of burn care in the USA was the development of effective topical antibacterial agents.

The use of topical drugs to reduce or eliminate bacteria on burns and other wounds has been practiced for years. Tannic acid was used in the early part of this century and almost universally discontinued by the 1940s due to systemic toxicity and the possible effect of further damaging partially destroyed skin.

In the 1940s and 1950s there was emphasis on the careful handling of burned and injured tissue, which led to the utilization of two techniques in burn care:

1) exposure, where burn wounds were exposed to the atmosphere until partial thickness wounds healed or when the eschar of full thickness wounds sloughed and the granulation tissue grafted;

2) utilization of compression dressings with a non-adherent material (often vaseline gauze) placed next to the wound, followed by bulky material held in place with a compression bandage. These dressings were changed as necessary until the partial thickness wounds healed and until the eschar of full thickness wounds was removed and grafts applied.

Wounds treated by these methods were susceptible to the development of local and systemic sepsis. This led to the search and development of topical antibacterial agents that would significantly reduce or eliminate bacteria on wounds without damaging composed skin or other delicate tissues.

One of the first agents developed for this purpose was sulfamylon cream by Dr. Robert Lindberg at Surgical Research Unit, now the U.S. Army Institute for Surgical Research at Ft. Sam Houston, Texas. The early clinical work was performed by Dr. John Moncrief.

About the same time, Dr. Carl Moyer and his colleagues advocated the use of dilute silver nitrate (0.05%). Sulfamylon cream could be used by the exposure technique or with the use of dressings, while the silver nitrate could be used only with dressings.

The development of other topical agents followed and one of the most popular was silver sulfadiazine. Others combined the use of agents such as silver and cerium, looking for the most effective agents. There is little question that topical antibacterial agents have contributed to the reduction in the morbidity and mortality of burn patients.

One of the most challenging problems in burn care has been the permanent coverage of large full thickness injuries. To solve this problem there have been attempts to develop synthetic biological materials that would serve as material to cover or incorporate into the wound for permanent closure.

Two of the early investigators in this field were Dr. John Burke at the Shriners Burns Institute in Boston and Dr. Iannias at M.I.T. They used animal collagen material placed next to excised wounds and covered with a silastic material for approximately two weeks until the collagen adhered to the wound bed and autografts could be applied to the collagen.

Others working in this field have used homografts to serve as the dermal component, removing the epidermis mechanically to prevent the rejection process and covering the dermis with keratinocytes.

There are currently others working in this field using a variety and combination of techniques of dermal and epidermal materials to achieve permanent wound closure with non-autologous materials.

The latest directory of the American Burn Association lists some 185 institutions as burn centers, units and teams. Personnel of many of these facilities have made significant contributions to burn care. It is not possible to mention all of these institutions; however, I want to comment on four of these facilities.

The first is the U.S. Army Institute of Surgical Research (ISR) at Ft. Sam Houston, Texas. Personnel from this institute have made significant contributions to all phases of burn care. One of the early commanders of the unit was Dr. Curtis Artz, known to many of you. Another commander and great contributor to burn research and care was Col. John Moncrief. The current Commander and Director of the ISR is Col. Basil Pruitt, who has been affiliated with the ISR for approximately 30 years and has been one of the most outstanding contributors to burn care during that time. Dr. Pruitt is a participant in this meeting.

Three other facilities that have worked extensively with burn care and research during the past 30 years are the Shriners Burns Institutes in Galveston, Cinncinnati, and Boston.

The Galveston unit has been directed by some outstanding surgeons and investigators including Dr. Curtis Artz, Dr. Duane Larson, and currently by Dr. David Herndon, also a participant in this meeting.

The Cincinnati unit was initially directed by Dr. Bruce MacMillan, who worked in many areas of burn care and investigation. The current director is Dr. Glenn Warden. He has contributed to the basic and clinical work in many areas of burn and trauma surgery and was at the ISR during Dr. Pruitt's tenure as Commander. Another who has made significant contributions at the Cincinnati unit is Dr. J. Wesley Alexander, who will be speaking during this meeting.

The third Shriners Burn Unit is in Boston. Its first director was Dr. John Burke, who was previously mentioned under the discussion of synthetic skin. The current director is Dr. Ron Tompkins, who has a broad interest in burn care and a special interest in metabolism and organ failure. Personnel from the Boston unit have made many other contributions to burns, especially in the areas of early excision and wound closure.

Author's adress:
John Boswick, MD
2005 Franklin St. # 355
Denver, CO 80205
USA

*Pathologie und Pathophysiologie
des Verbrennungstraumas*

Cause of mortality in thermally injured patients

W. G. Cioffi, S. H. Kim, B. A. Pruitt Jr

US Army Institute of Surgical Research, Houston

Concomitant with a decreasing mortality rate, a marked change in the cause of death has occurred in thermally injured patients over the last decade. In 1979, a mortality rate of 27.1% was observed in 273 patients admitted to this Institute. Between the years of 1987 und 1991, an overall mortality rate of 8.5% was observed in 1094 patients with a generally comparable age and burn size distribution compared to the 1979 cohort (Table 1). In 1979, infection was identified as the primary cause of death in 64% of patients, a figure which has declined to 42% over the past 5 years. In 1979, the mean postburn day of death was postburn day 24, but it has recently increased to postburn day 32.

Of the 1094 patients admitted to this Institute between January 1987 and December 1991, 93 patients died. The mean age of the nonsurvivors was 49 ± 2.6 years with a mean total burn size of $56.7\% \pm 2.5\%$. Inhalation injury diagnosed by either bronchoscopy or Xenon scintigraphy was present in 60 of 93 nonsurvivors. Pneumonia occurred in 60% of the patients and was most commonly diagnosed in nonsurviving patients with inhalation injury. Pneumonia was diagnosed only when the following criteria were met: presence of fever, new infiltrate on chest roentgenogram, predominant organism in sputum culture and sputum leukocytosis (>25 WBC/hpf). An autopsy was obtained in 52 of the 93 patients (55.9%) (Table 2). The postburn

Table 1. Age and burn size distribution comparing 1979 and 1987–1991

TBSA	Age			
	<20	21–40	41–60	>60
<20	13.9/21.6*	13.2/26.0	8.0/7.3	1.8/4.7
21–40	5.5/5.7	10.6/9.7	4.0/3.6	1.8/2.4
41–60	5.1/2.6	11.7/6.0	2.2/1.6	3.3/1.3
61–80	1.4/0.5	4.7/2.2	2.5/1.0	0.7/0.36
>80	1.4/0.3	4.7/1.6	1.8/0.8	0.35/0.4

* = Percent of total admissions 1979/1987–1991

Table 2. Demographics of nonsurvivors (1987–1991) N=93

Age	49.6 ± 2.6 years	(1–92 years)
TBSA	$56.7 \pm 2.5\%$	(0–99%)
Inhalation injury	64.5%	
Pneumonia	60%	
PBD Death	31.6 ± 4.4 days	(0–270 days)
Autopsy	55.9%	

Table 3. Mortality predictor

- $A = 6.026$
  $B = 0.1311 \cdot TBSA$
  $C = 0.2525 \cdot Age$
  $D = 0.7422 \cdot Age^2$
  $E = 0.4203 \cdot Age^3/10\,000$
- $F = A + B - C + D - E$
- $MORT = EXP(F)/1 + EXP(F)$
- Based upon all patients 1984–1988

day of death ranged from 0 to 270, with a mean of 31.6±4.4 days. Estimated mortality of the 93 nonsurvivors, using a predictor based upon age and burn size and developed using patient data between the years 1984 to 1988 was 62±3.6% (Table 3). Analysis of the cause of death in these 93 patients reveals deficiencies associated with burn-related mortality predictors based upon only age and burn size. Such predictors fail to account for the impact of pre-existing disease and other morbidity-related factors not directly related to the burn. When a predictor which accounts for the co-morbid effect of inhalation injury and pneumonia on outcome was used, estimated mortality for this cohort of patients was 76%. The median estimated mortality per patient was 0.897, indicating that the majority of patients had a very high likelihood of dying. Still, the co-morbid effects of pre-existing disease are not accounted for, and some patients with severe pre-existing cardiac or hepatic disease will be projected to have a low likelihood of not surviving.

Twelve of the 93 nonsurviving patients were resuscitation failures. Hemodynamic and pulmonary stability could not be achieved in these patients. Their ages ranged from 2 to 77 years, with a mean age of 35.4 years. Not surprisingly, they had a large mean burn size (82.7±4.2%). Ten of the 12 patients had a burn size in excess of 80%. The two patients with a burn size less than 80% TBSA both had severe inhalation injury, which added significantly to the difficulty in resuscitating these patients. The predicted mortality of these 12 patients was 93% with a range from 80 to 98%. These patients died, on average, on postburn day 2, with a range of 0 to 5 days.

Ten patients died from cardiac disease. Their average age was 60.4 years with a range of 1 to 91 years. The average burn size was 46.8%, with five of the 10 patients having inhalation injury. Pneumonia occurred in four of the 10 patients. Seven of the patients had a acute myocardial infarction, two had autopsy-documented severe cardiomyopathy, and one 3-month-old child sustained a cardiopulmonary arrest without apparent cause. The predicted mortality in this group of patients was 75%. The mean postburn day of death was 16.5 days and ranged from one to 70 days.

Pulmonary failure was the primary cause of death in 22 of the 93 nonsurvivors. Their mean age was 32.8±4.8 years, with a range of 1 to 69 years. Mean burn size was 62.6% (range 40–86% TBSA). Eighteen of the 22 patients had inhalation injury, and all 18 of these patients developed pneumonia. Of the four remaining patients, three had severe inhalation injury and died early in their postburn course prior to the development of pneumonia, and one patient died from a cardiopulmonary arrest secondary to an accidental extubation. The mean postburn time of death was 26.3 days and ranged from 0 to 120 days. The predicted mortality in this group of patients was 58%. This low predicted mortality indicates the failure of predictors based only on age and burn size to take into consideration the co-morbid effect of inhalation injury and pneumonia on outcome. When a predictor based upon age, burn size, and the presence of inhalation injury and pneumonia was used, the predicted mortality was 83%.

Ten patients died from multiple organ failure (MOF) without an identifiable septic focus. Multiple organ failure were defined according to strict clinical criteria and a minimum of three failed systems was required to assign this as the cause of death.

1) Respiratory failure as defined by Fulton and Jones which, in general, requires at least 120 h of mechanical respiratory support.
2) Cardiac failure based on the criteria of Tilney, which included a cardiac index (CI) of ≤ 2.2, cardiogenic shock requiring pressor support in combination with elevated pulmonary artery wedge pressures, arrhythmias not metabolic in origin that compromise cardiac output, or electrocardiogram (ECG) and enzyme evidence of perioperative myocardial infarction.
3) Hepatic failure defined as a bilirubin greater than 2 mg/dl with elevation of liver enzymes to levels twice normal.
4) Gastrointestinal failure defined as bleeding stress ulcers requiring at least two units of blood in 24 h.
5) Neurological failure defined as failure to respond to other than painful stimuli, or all grades of coma.
6) Renal failure defined as elevation of BUN and creatinine values of twice baseline levels.

The mean age of the MOF patients was 69.7 years (range 35–92 years). The mean burn size of this group was 45% (0–90% TBSA). The patient without thermal injury who died of multiple organ failure was a 75-year-old female with severe inhalation injury. Six of these 10 patients had inhalation injury and nine of the 10 developed pneumonia which was treated during their postburn course. The mean postburn day of death was 52.7 days and ranged from 9 to 166 days. The predicted mortality in this group of patients was 61% using the first predictor and 87% with the second.

Sepsis accounted for 21 of the 93 deaths. Sepsis was defined as the presence of positive blood cultures in the clinical setting of hypotension, decreased systemic vascular resistance, and increased cardiac index. The mean age of this group of patients was 59.1 ± 4.1 years and ranged from 28 to 88 years. The mean burn size was $62.4 \pm 5\%$. Thirteen of the 21 patients sustained inhalation injury, and pneumonia was present in 17 of the 21 patients. The predicted mortality for this group was 85% using the second predictor. In 13 of the 21 patients the origin of sepsis was clearly pulmonary, with 12 bacterial and one candidal pneumonia diagnosed. One patient with bacterial pneumonia also had bilateral adrenal infarction found at autopsy. Of the remaining eight patients, six had an identifiable source of sepsis: two patients with necrotizing enterocolitis, one patient with klebsiella wound infection and bilateral adrenal infarction, one patient with a gram-negative subacute bacterial endocarditis, one patient with subacute staphylococcal endocarditis, and one patient with fungemia secondary to fungal burn wound invasion. Two patients had gram-negative sepsis without an identifiable primary source at autopsy.

Neurologic complications accounted for seven of the 93 deaths. The mean age of this group was 42.7 ± 12.1 years, and the mean burn size $36 \pm 7.5\%$. Four elderly patients sustained a CVA at or shortly after the time of their injury and eventually succumbed from their cerebrovascular accident. One patient with significant head trauma and relatively minor burns died from his head injury. One patient died from cerebral hypoxia secondary to asphyxiant inhalation at the scene of the fire. One patient died of cerebral edema of an unknown etiology.

Fulminant hepatic failure was responsible for three deaths. All three patients were middle-aged males with significant ethyl alcohol abuse histories. All had significant hepatic disease prior to injury. Their mean age was 51.7 ± 1.8 years, and mean burn size $29 \pm 4.8\%$. The mean predicted mortality for this small group of patients was 5%. It must be noted that the predictor does not take into consideration pre-existent disease such as hepatic failure.

One patient of the 93 died from a pulmonary embolus. This was a 63-year-old morbidly obese female with a 30% TBSA burn, inhalation injury, and pneumonia. This patient sustained a massive pulmonary embolus on postburn day 30 despite heparin prophylaxis at an infusion level sufficient to maintain a partial thromboplastin time between 40 and 50 s.

Four patients died from aspiration. Three of the four patients had pre-existing psychiatric disease, and all three died from immediate cardiopulmonary arrest. One patient developed prolonged respiratory failure following aspiration of gastric contents and eventually died of pulmonary failure. At autopsy numerous staphylococcal pulmonary abscesses were identified. The mean age of this group of patients was 48 years and mean burn size was 41%.

Two patients died from massive adrenal infarction documented at autopsy, but not diagnosed premortem. Neither patient had systemic sepsis at the time of death. The first was a 25-year-old male with an 89% burn who died on postburn day 12. The second was a 41-year-old male with a 64.5% burn who died on postburn day 20. Both patients had sustained inhalation injury and had documented pneumonia which was treated with appropriate antibiotics. At autopsy, no discernable cause for adrenal infarction could be found.

Despite our ability to resuscitate the majority of patients from their initial injury, 13% of the deaths in the past 5 years were secondary to our inability to achieve cardiopulmonary stability in the first 2 postburn days. Despite the decline in infection as a cause of death in burn patients, it is still the leading cause of demise in thermally injured patients. As is apparent from this review, the focus of infection has shifted from the burn wound to the lung. Of the 47 infection-related deaths which occurred in 1979, the focus of infection was the lung in 28 (59.6%) and the wound in 12 (25.5%). Between 1987 and 1991, the lung was the primary focus in 79.8% of 39 patients who died of infection. The wound accounted for only 5.1% of infection-

Table 4. Mortality (1979) segregated by age and burn size

TBSA	Age			
	<20	21–40	41–60	>60
<20	0%	0%	0%	40%
21–40	6.6%	0%	36%	60%
41–60	21.4%	18.7%	50%	77%
61–80	75%	77%	100%	100%
>80	100%	100%	100%	100%

Table 5. Mortality (1987–1991) segregated by age and burn size

TBSA	Age			
	<20	21–40	41–60	>60
<20	0.4%	0%	2.5%	11.5%
21–40	0%	0.9%	15.4%	34.6%
41–60	24.1%	7.6%	33.3%	80%
61–80	0%	12.5%	60%	100%
>80	75%	72.2%	75%	75%

related deaths. Inhalation injury and subsequent pneumonia are still significant co-morbid factors. Survival rates have significantly improved over the past decade, especially in mid-size burns (40–80 % TBSA) in middle aged adults (20–60 years) (Tables 4, 5). The improvement in survival is related to many changes in patient care, including infection control, burn wound excision, nutritional care and, most recently, the use of high-frequency ventilation in patients with inhalation injury. Not surprisingly, pre-existing cardiac, neurologic, and hepatic disease may have significant co-morbid effects on outcome, especially in the elderly. The gradual lenghtening of the mean post burn day of death over the past decade reflects the improved level of critical care which is applied to critically ill severely burned patients. Despite this improvement, failure to obtain prompt wound closure in patients with massive thermal injury places them at risk for development of late complications, principally infection, which adversely affect outcome.

References

References available from the author.

Author's address:
W. G. Cioffi, M.D.
US Army Institute of Surgical Research
Fort Sam Houston
Texas 78234-5012
USA

Pathologie und Pathophysiologie des Verbrennungstraumas

K. Wegener

Pathologisches Institut des Klinikums Ludwigshafen/Rh.

Todesursachen bei 466 obduzierten Verbrennungspatienten zwischen 1972 und 1991

In den Jahren von 1972 bis 1991 sind im Pathologischen Institut des Klinikums Ludwigshafen etwas mehr als 500 Verstorbene der Verbrennungsklinik Ludwigshafen obduziert worden.

Von 466 dieser Patienten – 387 Männern und 79 Frauen – liegen so ausführliche Daten vor, daß wir Korrelationen zwischen den Parametern „Todesursache" auf der einen Seite und „Geschlecht", „Alter", „Krankheitsdauer" und anderen auf der Gegenseite haben herstellen können. Über die verschiedenen Todesursachen, ihre Definitionen und ihre Korrelationen mit anderen Parametern bei den 466 obduzierten Patienten will ich sprechen.

Abbildung 1 zeigt die Häufigkeitsverteilung der Todesfälle über verschiedene Altersgruppen. Auf der x-Achse die Altersgruppen von 0 bis 90 Jahren, auf der y-Achse die Zahl verstorbener Patienten. Die hellen Säulen geben die Häufigkeiten für die Männer, die dunklen für die Frauen an. Der Altersgipfel bei den Männern liegt zwischen 30 und 40 Jahren, er zeigt einen steilen Anstieg und Abfall, bedingt dadurch, daß es sich bei diesen Patienten vorwiegend um Männer im berufsfähigen

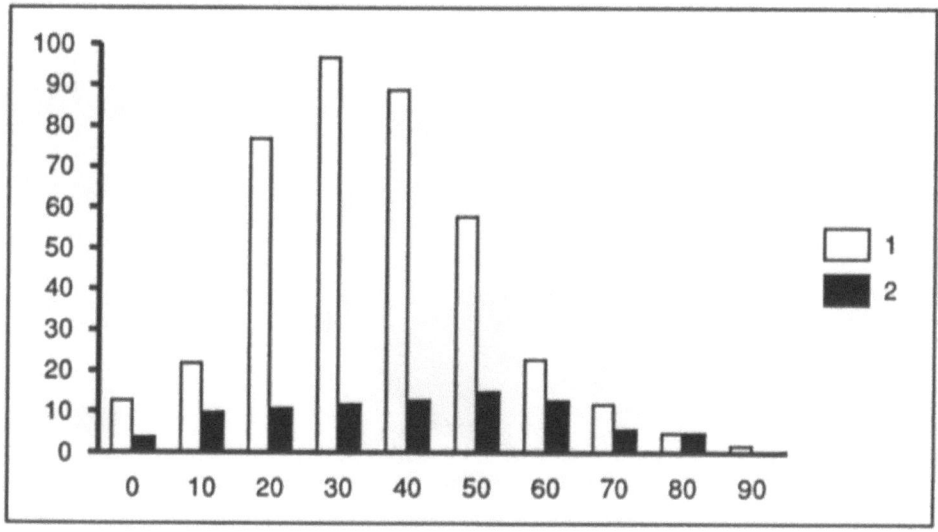

Abb. 1. Altersverteilung der Verstorbenen (1 = Männer; 2 = Frauen)

Tabelle 1. Todesursachen

1. Multiorganversagen
2. Rechtsherzversagen
3. Sepsis
4. Energetisch-dynamische Herzinsuffizienz
5. Linksherzversagen
6. Zentraler Tod
7. Bronchopneumonie
8. Todesursache nicht definierbar

Alter handelt. Eine vergleichbare Verteilung fehlt bei den Frauen, sie erleiden ihre Verbrennungen vorwiegend durch häusliche Unfälle.

Wir haben 8 Todesursachen unterschieden (Tabelle 1). In allen Fällen war „Verbrennung, Verbrühung oder Verätzung" das Grundleiden und eine dieser Diagnosen die sogenannte mittelbare Todesursache.

Die mittelbare Todesursache gibt den Prozess an, der im Verlaufe der Verbrennungskrankheit den Umschlag von der allgemeinen Katabiose in die Anabiose verhindert, also den Punkt markiert, von dem an es für den Patienten kein „Zurück" mehr gibt. Die Todesursache *Multiorganversagen* ist von uns diagnostiziert worden in den Fällen, in denen klinische und patho-anatomische Schockzeichen bestanden haben und keine Sepsis vorgelegen hat. Entsprechendes gilt für die Todesursache *Bronchopneumonie*. Für die Todesursache Sepsis haben wir klinische Zeichen, positive Blutkultur, große bunte Organe oder septische Metastasen verlangt. In den Fällen eines septischen Schocks haben wir die Todesursache *Sepsis* beibehalten. Die Todesursache *Rechtsherzversagen* betrifft Patienten mit fulminanter Lungenarterienembolie. Von *Linksherzversagen* haben wir gesprochen, wenn es im Verlaufe der

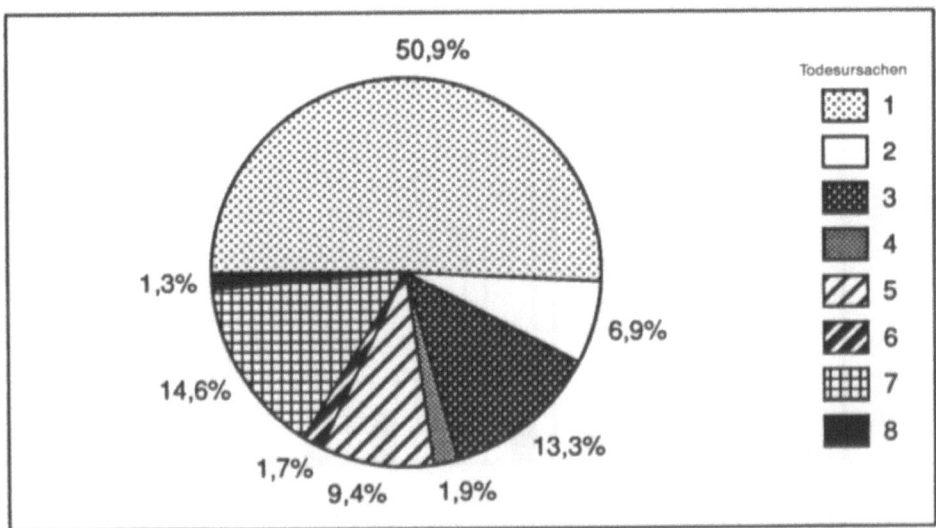

Abb. 2. Prozentuale Verteilung der Todesursachen bei allen Verstorbenen

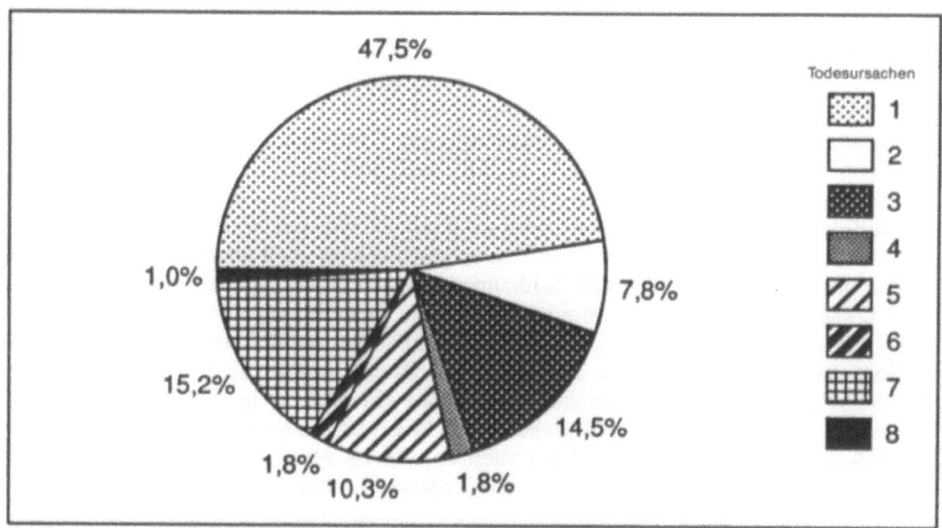

Abb. 3. Prozentuale Verteilung der Todesursachen bei Männern

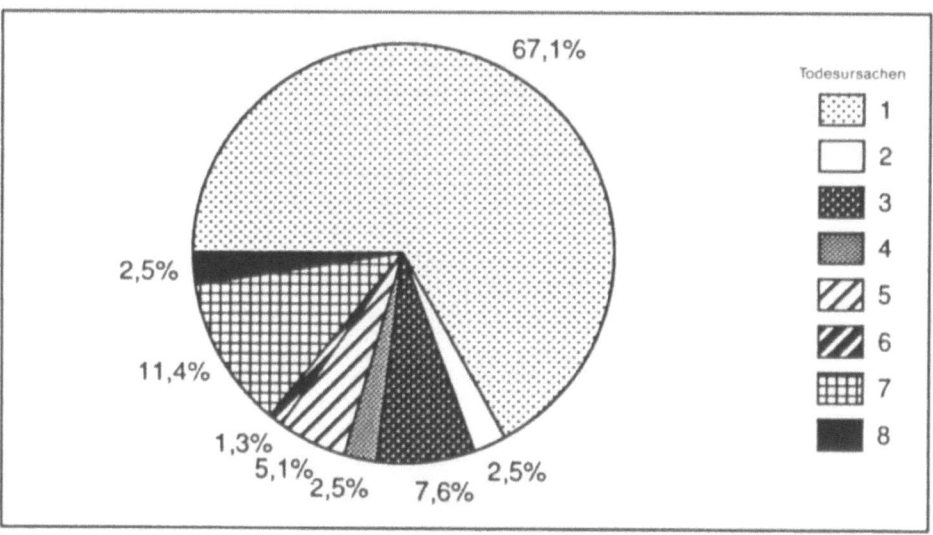

Abb. 4. Prozentuale Verteilung der Todesursachen bei Frauen

Verbrennungskrankheit zu hypoxischen Schäden am Herzen gekommen ist. In allen diesen Fällen hat ein Vorschaden in Form einer Koronarsklerose oder einer Linksherzhypertrophie bestanden. Von *zentralem Tod* haben wir in Fällen von Hirnkontusionen und intrakraniellen Blutungen gesprochen. Die Todesursache *energetisch dynamische Herzinsuffizienz* betrifft Fälle mit Hyperkaliämie, Hypokaliämie oder Hypernatriämie. Die Abbildung 2 zeigt die prozentuale Verteilung der einzelnen Todesursachen im Gesamtkollektiv: In 50% sterben die Patienten im Multiorganversagen, in 6,9% am Rechtsherzversagen, in 13,3% an der Sepsis, in 1,9% an der energetisch dynamischen Herzinsuffizienz, in 9,4% am Linksherzversagen, in 1,7% an einem zentralen Tod, in 14,6% an der Bronchopneumonie und in 1,3% war die Todesursache nicht eindeutig bestimmbar.

Betrachtet man die prozentuale Verteilung der Todesursachen getrennt für Männer (Abb. 3) und Frauen (Abb. 4), so fällt auf, daß signifikant mehr Frauen im Multiorganversagen versterben als Männer und die Zahl der tödlichen Lungenarterienembolien bei Männern etwa 3mal so hoch ist wie bei Frauen. Die Zahl der tödlichen Sepsisfälle dagegen ist bei Frauen nur halb so groß als bei Männern. Das gleiche gilt für die Todesursache Linksherzversagen. Hingegen die Häufigkeit der Todesursache Bronchopneumonie ist bei beiden Geschlechtern fast gleich.

Im Verlaufe der Verbrennungskrankheit sind bestimmte Zeitabschnitte besonders wichtig: der erste Tag, die erste und die zweite Woche und die Zeit nach der zweiten Woche. Die Abbildung 5 zeigt die prozentuale Häufigkeit der Todesursachen bei Patienten, die am ersten Tag verstorben sind. Die Abbildung 6 zeigt die prozentuale Häufigkeit von Todesursachen bei Patienten, die in der ersten Woche verstorben sind. Von den 58 Patienten, die am ersten Tage verstorben sind, sind 48 oder 82,9% im Multiorganversagen verstorben, 6,9% im Linksherzversagen. Die übrigen Todesursachen spielen prozentual keine Rolle. Diese hohe Prozentzahl für die Todesursache „Multiorganversagen" hängt damit zusammen, daß es sich bei einem großen Teil dieser Verstorbenen um Patienten mit schwersten Verbrennungen und/oder relevanten Begleitverletzungen gehandelt hat, bei denen wegen der infausten Prognose keine Maximaltherapie durchgeführt worden ist. In der ersten Woche dagegen ist die Zahl der Todesfälle an Multiorganversagen bei den 129 Patienten dieses Teilkollektivs deutlich zurückgegangen. 17,1% der Patienten sind an Bronchopneumonie und 7,8% an Linksherzversagen gestorben.

Bei den 136 Patienten, die in der zweiten Woche nach der Verbrennung verstorben sind, tritt das Multiorganversagen nur noch in 46,8% der Fälle auf. Mit 19,6% steht

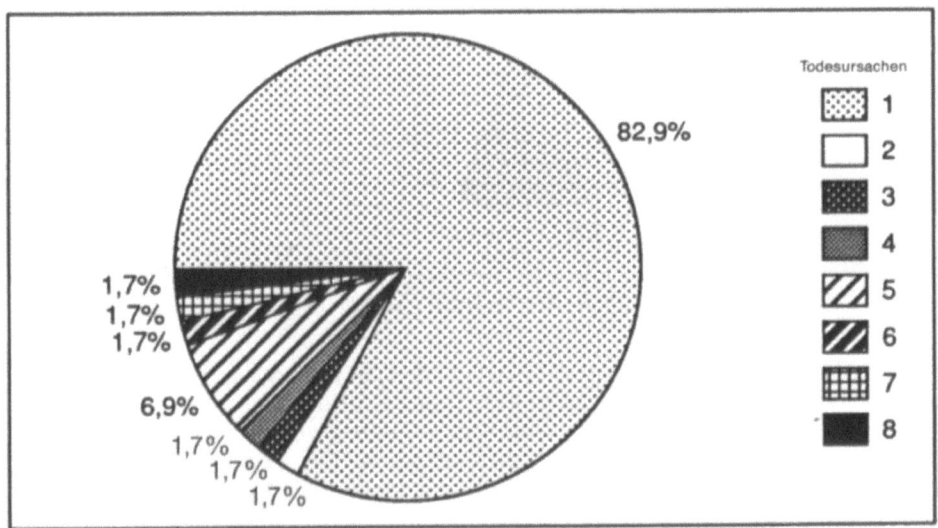

Abb. 5. Relative Häufigkeit von Todesursachen bei Patienten, die am 1. Tag verstarben

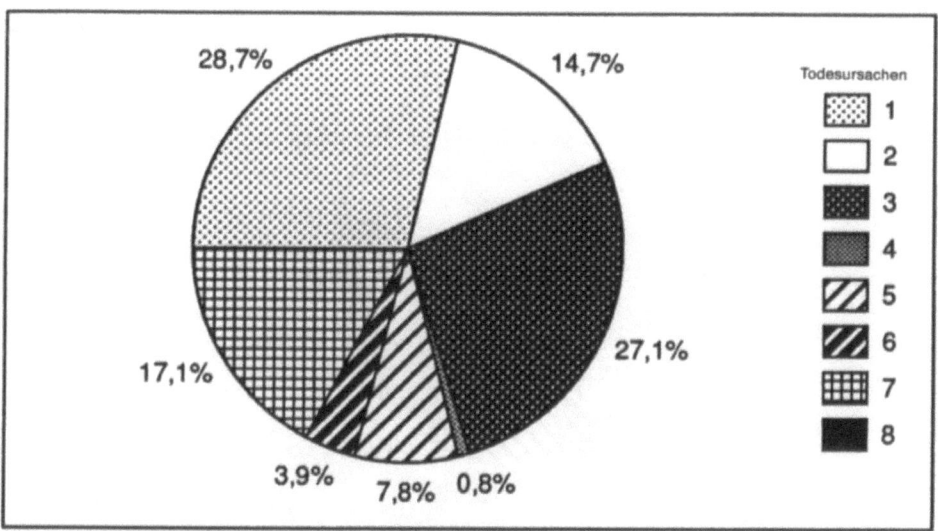

Abb. 6. Relative Häufigkeit von Todesursachen bei Patienten, die in der 1. Woche starben

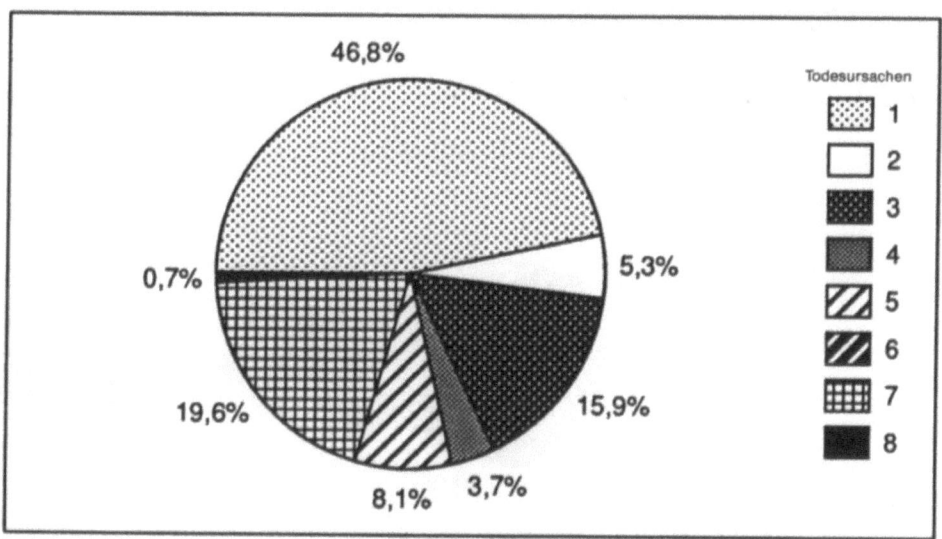

Abb. 7. Relative Häufigkeit von Todesursachen bei Patienten, die in der 2. Woche starben

die Bronchopneumonie an zweiter Stelle, und mit 15,9% die Sepsis an 3. Stelle der Todesursachen (Abb. 7). Nach der zweiten Woche sterben nur noch etwa ein Drittel aller Patienten am Multiorganversagen, 14,7% am Rechtsherzversagen durch Lungenarterienembolien, fast ein Drittel an der Sepsis – das sind fast genauso viele wie am Multiorganversagen – und 17% an der Bronchopneumonie. Das bedeutet, daß sich die beiden wichtigen Komplikationen: Sepsis und Bronchopneumonie mit der Länge des Krankheitslagers als Todesursachen immer mehr in den Vordergrund schieben.

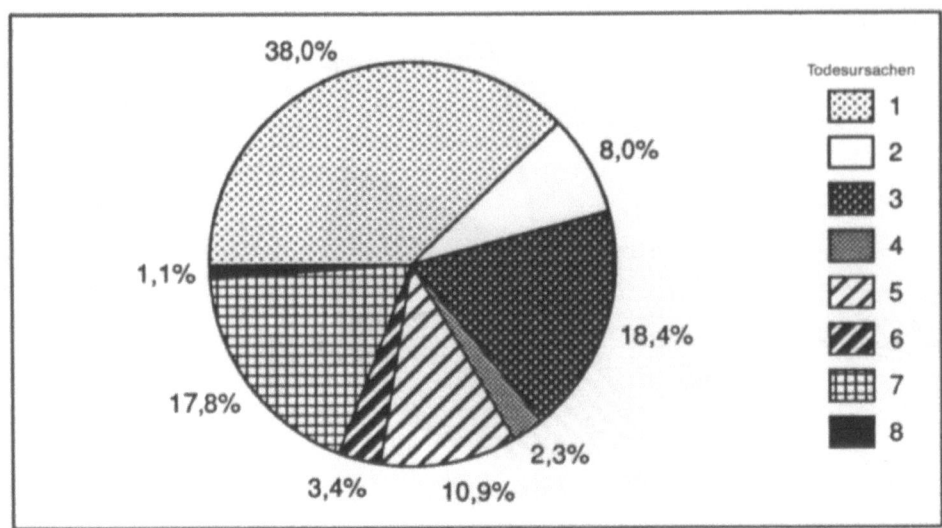

Abb. 8. Prozentuale Verteilung der Todesursachen bei Verstorbenen mit ≦40% verbrannter KOF

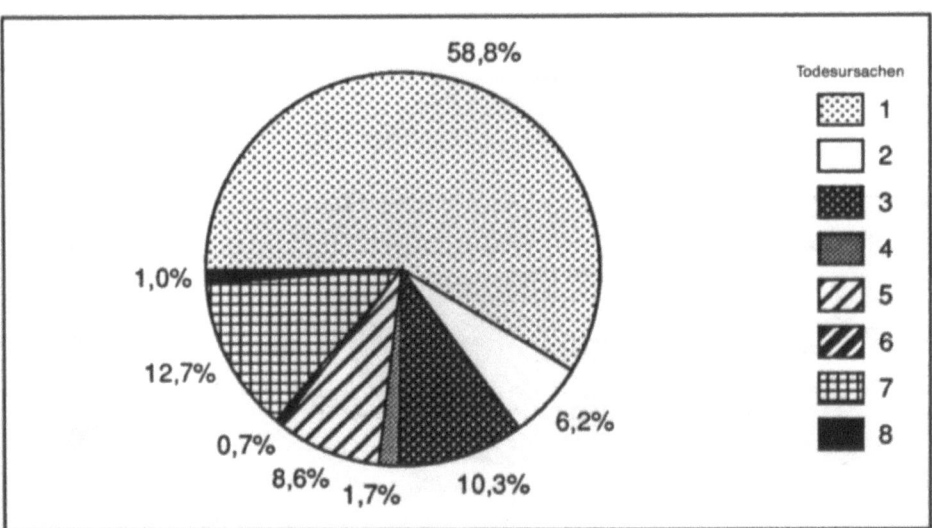

Abb. 9. Prozentuale Verteilung der Todesursachen bei Verstorbenen mit >40% verbrannter KOF

Eine weitere interessante Korrelation zeigen die beiden nächsten Diagramme. Abbildung 8 zeigt die prozentuale Verteilung der Todesursachen bei Patienten mit weniger als 40% verbrannter Körperoberfläche. Abbildung 9 zeigt die Todesursachenverteilung bei mehr als 40% verbrannter Körperoberfläche. Es ist deutlich, daß die Schwererverbrannten signifikant häufiger am Multiorganversagen sterben als die weniger Verbrannten. Dagegen ist bei den weniger stark Verbrannten die Todesursache Sepsis fast doppelt so häufig wie bei den schwerer Verbrannten. Ähnliches gilt

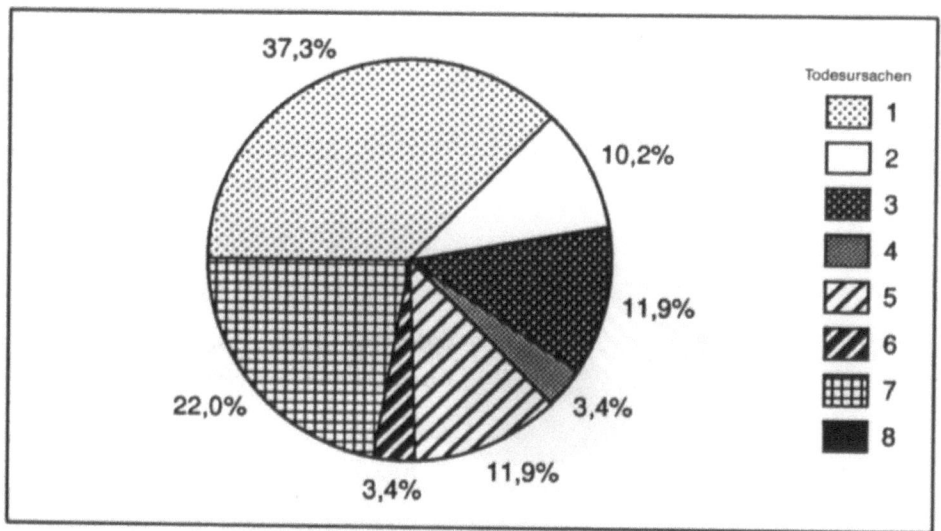

Abb. 10. Relative Häufigkeit von Todesursachen bei Patienten mit Verbrennungen II°

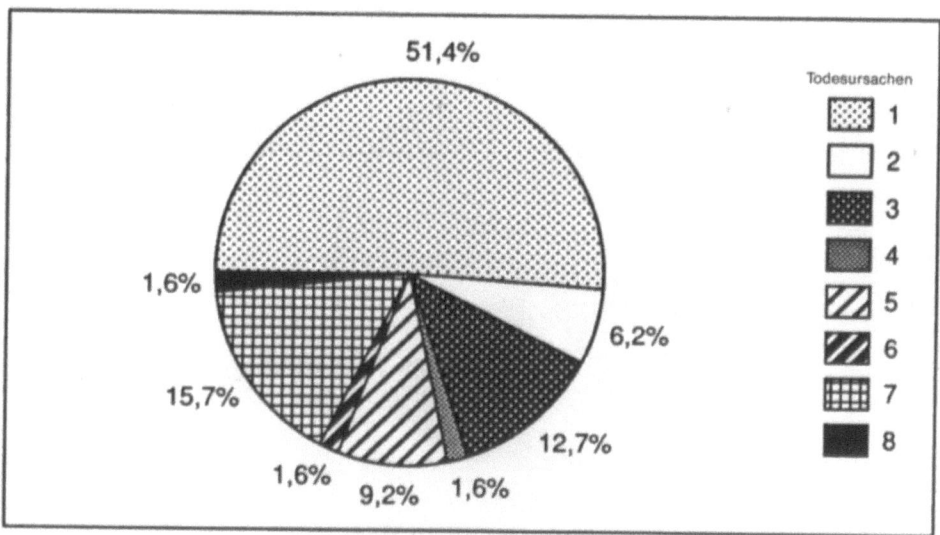

Abb. 11. Prozentuale Verteilung der Todesursachen bei Patienten mit Verbrennungen II–III°

für die Bronchopneumonie, die in 17,8% die Todesursache bei den weniger stark Verbrannten und in 12,7% bei den stärker verbrannten Patienten darstellt.

Betrachtet man die Korrelation zwischen Todesursachen und der Schwere der Verbrennung, so wird folgendes deutlich: Ein Drittel aller zweitgradig verbrannten Patienten stirbt am Schock, 10,2% sterben an einer Lungenarterienembolie, fast 12% an einer Sepsis, genauso viele im Linksherzversagen, 22% an der Bronchopneumonie (Abb. 10).

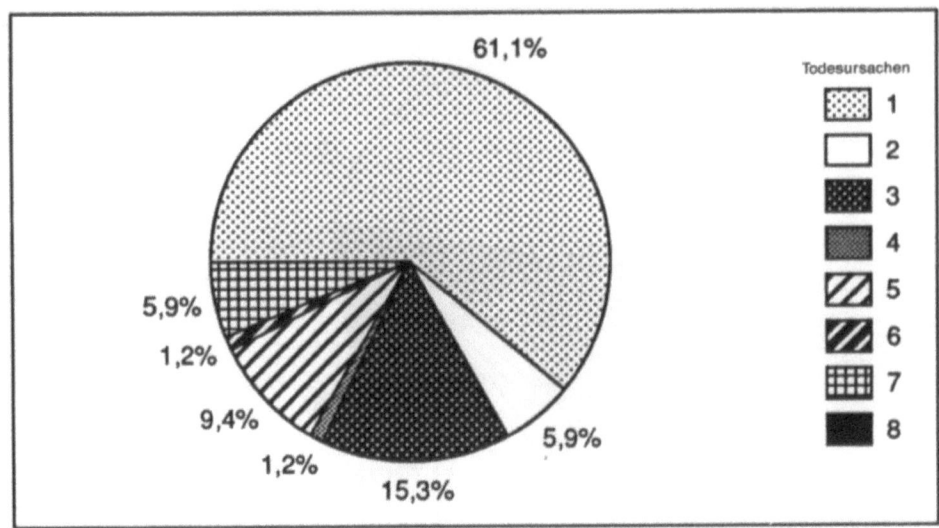

Abb. 12. Prozentuale Verteilung der Todesursachen bei Patienten mit Verbrennungen III°

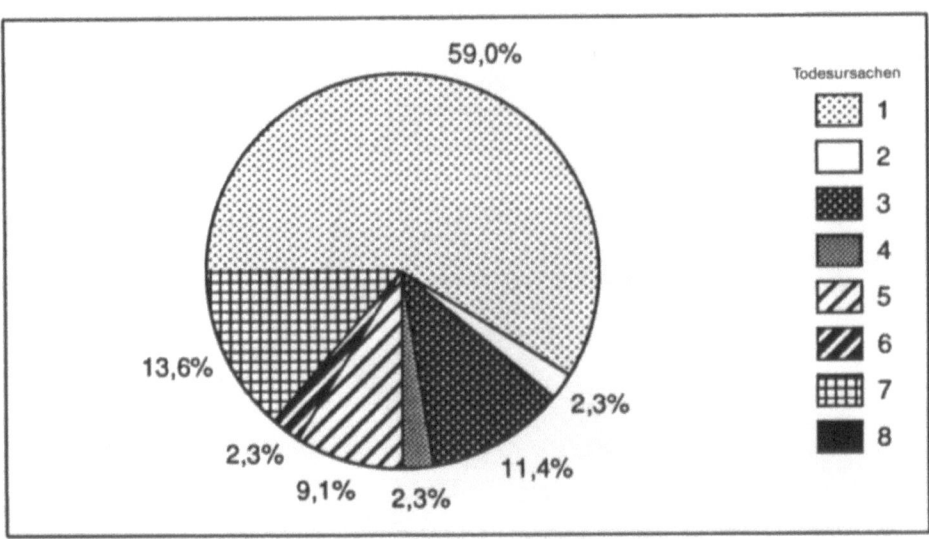

Abb. 13. Relative Häufigkeit der Todesursachen in den einzelnen Altersgruppen

Ganz anders liegen die Verhältnisse bei Patienten mit zweit- bis drittgradiger (Abb. 11) und drittgradiger Verbrennung (Abb. 12). Mit der Schwere der Verbrennung nimmt der prozentuale Anteil der Todesursache Multiorganversagen deutlich zu, von etwa 37% über 51,4% auf 61,1%. Die Todesursache Sepsis steigt nur geringgradig an, die Todesursache Bronchopneumonie nimmt deutlich ab. Dies bedeutet, daß die Todesursache Multiorganversagen gegenüber der Todesursache Bronchopneumonie mit Zunahme der Schwere der Verbrennung an Gewicht gewinnt.

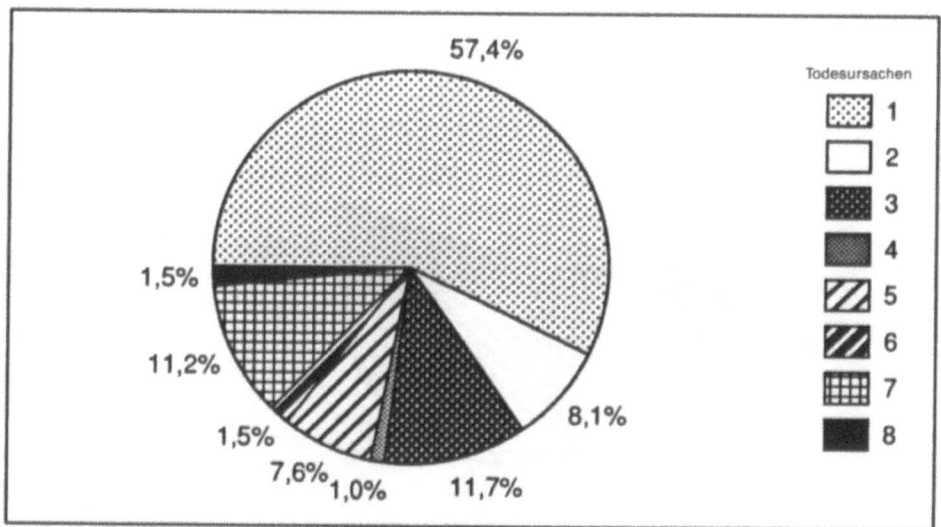

Abb. 14. Relative Häufigkeit der Todesursachen in den einzelnen Altersgruppen

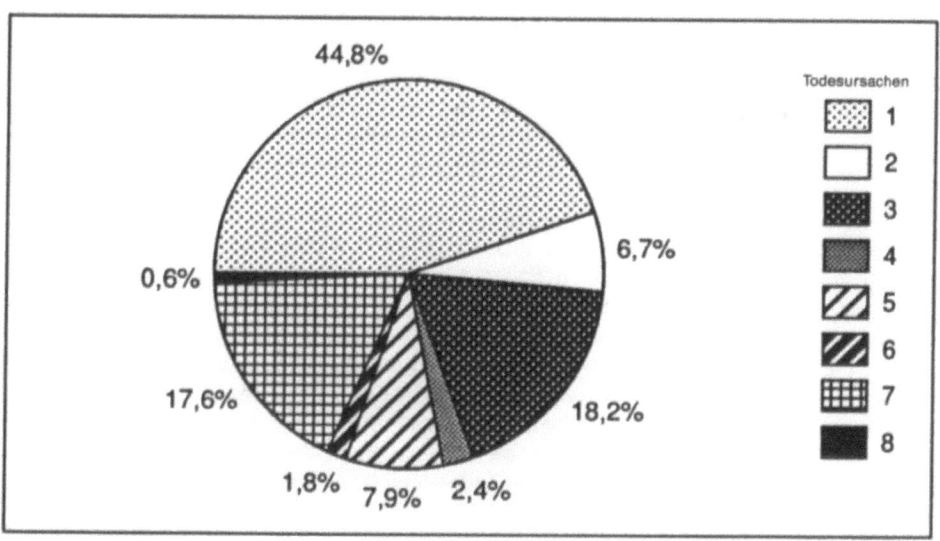

Abb. 15. Relative Häufigkeit der Todesursachen in den einzelnen Altersgruppen

Eine letzte Korrelation sei betrachtet: In den beiden Altersgruppen der 6 bis 20-jährigen (Abb. 13) und 21 bis 40-jährigen (Abb. 14) Patienten führt die Todesursache Multiorganversagen oder Schock mit fast 60%, die Todesursache Sepsis ist in beiden Altersgruppen fast gleich häufig, gleiches gilt für die Todesursachen Bronchopneumonie und Linksherzversagen.

Ganz anders sind die Verhältnisse in der Altersgruppe der 40 bis 60-jährigen (Abb. 15) und der älter als 60 Jahre alten Patienten (Abb. 16): Hier ist die Todesursa-

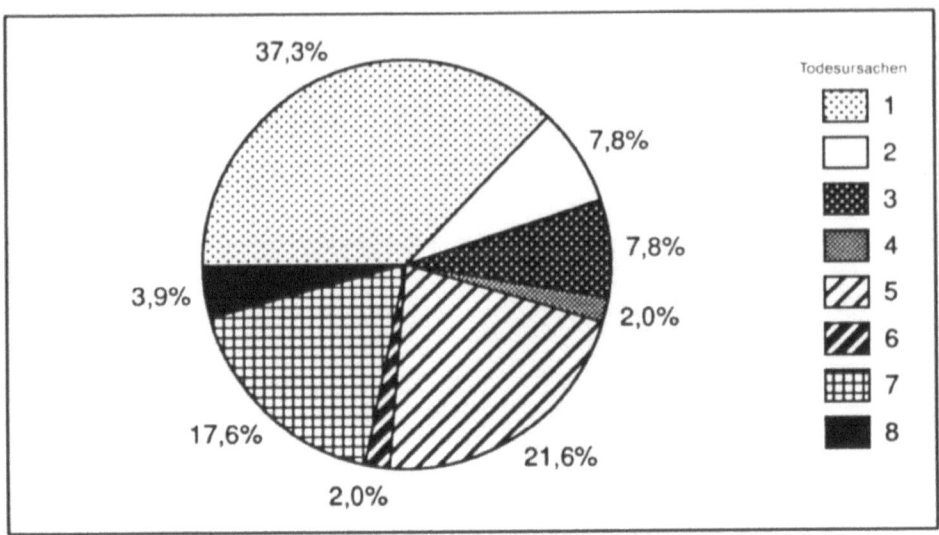

Abb. 16. Relative Häufigkeit der Todesursachen in den einzelnen Altersgruppen

che Multiorganversagen zurückgegangen. Bei den 40 bis 60-jährigen steigt die Zahl der Sepsisfälle deutlich an, wie auch die der Pneumonien. Und bei den 60 Jahre und älteren Patienten kommt es in fast einem Viertel aller Fälle zum Tod im Linksherzversagen, die Bronchopneumonie bleibt an Häufigkeit gleich, die Fälle von Sepsis gehen deutlich zurück.

Ich kehre zum Anfang meines Vortrages, zur Häufigkeit der einzelnen Todesursachen zurück. Was sagt ein Vergleich unserer Daten mit denen der Literatur? Tabelle 2 zeigt einzelne Todesursachen in Prozent, wie sie verschiedene Autoren in ihren Arbeiten angegeben haben. Sie sehen die großen Unterschiede zum Beispiel der Todesursache Sepsis: Bei Algöwer 16,7%, bei Arturson 34,2%, bei Feller 48,3%, bei Glor 18,6%, bei Grötzinger nur 8,5%. Desweiteren bemerken sie, daß die Todesursache „akutes Nierenversagen" bei Arturson, Glor und Grötzinger nicht unbeträchtliche Prozentsätze ausmacht, daß aber Algöwer und Feller diese Todesursache gar nicht angeben. Ähnlich steht es mit der Todesursache Bronchopneumonie, die bei Arturson nicht erscheint. Oder mit der Todesursache Herzkreislaufversagen, die nur Arturson und Grötzinger benutzen.

Analysiert man die Daten über Todesursachen in der Literatur, vergleicht sie mit den eigenen, und versucht zu ergründen, wodurch die zum Teil erheblichen Diskrepanzen zustandekommen, so läßt sich festhalten:

1. Prozentzahlen dieser Art haben nur einen Sinn, wenn der Begriff „Todesursache" genau definiert ist.
2. In der Literatur erscheinen eine ganze Reihe von Todesursachen, die nicht benutzt werden sollten, wie zum Beispiel Herz-Kreislauf-Versagen. Dieser Begriff sagt nicht viel aus. Wichtig wäre, Kliniker und Pathologen könnten sich auf eine umschriebene Gruppe verschiedener Todesursachen einigen und mit diesen Begriffen arbeiten.

Tabelle 2. Todesursachen

Autor	Todesursachen					
	Schock	Sepsis	Broncho-pneumonie	Akutes Nierenversagen	Herz-Kreislaufversagen	Sonstige
Allgöwer (1957)	8,3	16,7	25,0	–	–	50,0
Arturson (1964)	15,8	34,2	–	23,7	15,8	10,5
Feller (1964)	8,3	48,3	13,3	–	–	30,1
Gloor (1966)	10,4	18,6	20,8	12,5	–	37,7
Grözinger (1970)	3,4	8,5	11,9	18,6	15,2	42,4

3. Die Kollektive, an denen Aussagen über die Todesursachen und ihre Korrelationen gemacht werden, dürfen nicht zu klein sein, zu kleine Kollektive geben ein ungenaues Bild.
4. Nur eine Synopsis klinischer und pathoanatomischer Daten bieten die Gewähr, mit der Angabe einer bestimmten Todesursache der wahren Situation am nächsten zu kommen.
5. Aber auch wenn diese eben genannten Prämissen erfüllt sind, bedarf es für jedes Kollektiv einer eingehenden Diskussion, weil das Patientengut sich in ein und derselben Klinik mit wachsenden Therapieerfolgen stetig ändert und an den einzelnen Kliniken in Bezug auf Alter, Art der Verbrennung und andere Parameter differiert, die Therapien in den einzelnen Kliniken unterschiedlich sind, und weil über Pathogenese und Wertigkeit einzelner Kriterien unter Klinikern und Pathologen keine Einigkeit besteht. Ich nenne als Beispiel meines Faches nur die pulmonalen hyalinen Membranen, die von den einen als Äquivalent des Schocks im Sinne einer extravasalen Gerinnung, von den anderen als Folge der Beatmung mit Sauerstoff in hohen Konzentrationen angesehen werden.

Das Wichtigste ist: Wir müssen genaue Definitionen erarbeiten und wir müssen so viele Verstorbene wie irgend möglich obduzieren lassen.

Literatur

1. Allgöwer M, Siegrist J (1957) Verbrennungen. Springer-Verlag, Berlin, Göttingen, Heidelberg
2. Arturson G (1964) Analysis of 38 death from burns (1951–1962). Acta Chir Scand 128:25
3. Feller I, Hendrix RC (1964) Clinical pathological study of sixty fatally burned patients. Surg Gyn Obst 119:1
4. Gloor F (1966) Pathologisch-anatomische Befunde bei tödlichen Verbrennungen. Praxis: 211
5. Grözinger KH, Götz R (1970) Todesfälle nach thermischen Verletzungen. Monatsschr Unfallheilkd 73:197

Anschrift des Verfassers:
Prof. Dr. K. Wegener
Klinikum der Stadt Ludwigshafen
Pathologisches Institut
Bremserstr. 79
D-67063 Ludwigshafen-Oggersheim

Pathogenetische Mechanismen der verbrennungsinduzierten Immunsuppression

M. Köller, J. Brom und W. König

Lehrstuhl für Medizinische Mikrobiologie und Immunologie, Ruhr-Universität Bochum

Die Wiederherstellung und Aufrechterhaltung der kardiovaskulären und respiratorischen Funktionen, die spezielle Volumenersatztherapie, das frühzeitige Abtragen tief verbrannter Hautareale, die neuen Transplantationstechniken und die hochkalorische Ernährung haben die Überlebensrate schwerbrandverletzter Patienten in der frühen posttraumatischen Phase erheblich verbessert. In der späteren posttraumatischen Phase ist gerade diese Patientengruppe aber durch Infektion und Sepsis vital gefährdet. Das septische Syndrom mit fortschreitendem Multiorganversagen stellt heute das Hauptrisiko für den schwerbrandverletzten Patienten dar [6]. Epidemiologische Studien haben gezeigt, daß 60–80% aller spät auftretenden posttraumatischen Todesfälle auf Sepsis und damit verbundenem konsekutiven Multiorganversagen zurückgeführt werden können [36].

Die Infektion der Brandwunden

Das Spektrum der Keimbesiedlung von Verbrennungswunden hat sich in den letzten Jahrzehnten auch aufgrund des Selektionsdrucks durch die antibiotische Therapie deutlich verändert [28]. Eine grundlegende Veränderung der mikrobiell-induzierten Morbiditäts- und Mortalitätsrate ist damit aber nicht einhergegangen. Oft entwickelt sich unter dem permanenten Selektionsdruck durch die jeweilige kliniktypische Antibiotikatherapie auf Intensivstationen ein epidemisches Ansteigen von antibiotikaresistenten Stämmen. So berichteten wir für die Brandverletzten-Intensivstation der Bochumer Universitätsklinik „Bergmannsheil" über das präferentielle Auftreten von Staphylococcus aureus und Pseudomonas aeruginosa in den Brandwunden [41]. Durch die systematische Auswertung von Antibiogrammen wurde auch der hohe Anteil von multiresistenten Stämmen mit Mehrfachresistenzen gegen bis zu 16 verschiedenen Antibiotika dokumentiert [41]. Die Eintrittspforten der Mikroorganismen sind beim Brandverletzten primär die großflächigen offenen Wunden, aber natürlich auch die chirurgischen Maßnahmen und die invasive Patientenversorgung und -überwachung.

Neue experimentelle Daten sprechen außerdem für eine Translokation enteraler Mikroorganismen und bakterieller Toxine wie Endotoxin durch die intestinalen Mukosa-Schranken [2, 18].

Die Anflutung bakterieller Pathogenitätsfaktoren wie z.B. Endotoxine führt zu signifikanten Reaktionen der körpereigenen Abwehr. Eigene Untersuchungen haben gezeigt, daß viele bakterielle Toxine in der Lage sind, die Bildung von Entzündungsmediatoren zu induzieren und zu modulieren [7].

Wir konnten anhand klinischer Isolate von Verbrennungspatienten zeigen, daß unterschiedliche zellgebundene und lösliche Pathogenitätsfaktoren von P. aeruginosa-Stämmen (z.B. hitzelabile und hitzestabile Hämolysine) die Generierung von Entzündungsmediatoren wie Histamin oder Leukotrienen in definierter Weise beeinflussen [5]. Taxonomisch identische Stämme können diesbezüglich in ihrer Pathogenität deutlich variieren. So wiesen wir nach, daß die *in vitro*-Virulenz wundinfizierender Staphylokokken-Isolate von Schwerbrandverletzen sich in der Phase der Kolonisierung anders verhält als in der Phase der Invasion [43]. Im Vergleich zu den die Wundoberfläche besiedelnden Stämmen exprimieren invasive Staphylokokken vermehrt zellgebundene Pathogenitätsfaktoren (Toxine). Gleichzeitig ist jedoch ihre Freisetzung in löslicher Form vermindert. Invasive Stämme können offensichtlich durch Unterlaufen der lokalen Infektabwehr einen Selektionsvorteil entwickeln. Die Charakteristika der ausgedehnten thermischen Verletzung mit den großflächigen Wunden, die hohe Umgebungstemperatur und Luftfeuchtigkeit innerhalb der Intensivstation, das Auftreten von multiresistenten Bakterienstämmen, der Pathogenitätserwerb invasiver Mikroorganismen und auch die intensive Behandlung und Betreuung der Patienten durch das Klinikpersonal (Gefahr der Kreuzinfektion) sind Faktoren, die die mikrobielle Kolonisierung und Invasion fördern. Zusätzlich ist die körpereigene Infektabwehr der Verbrennungspatienten durch eine traumainduzierte Immunsuppression geschwächt. Mikrobielle Kolonisation und Immunsupression sind typische Elemente der entstehenden sogenannten „Verbrennungskrankheit", die sich gegenseitig bedingen und verstärken können. Unsere heutigen Vorstellungen über die pathogenetischen Zusammenhänge zwischen gestörter Infektabwehr und dem septischen Syndrom mit fortschreitendem Multiorganversagen konzentrieren sich auf ein „fehlgesteuertes" Immunsystem. Dabei spielen die hochpotenten löslichen Effektor-Elemente der spezifischen und unspezifischen Infektabwehr wie z.B. TNF-α oder Interleukin 6 eine entscheidende Rolle.

Septisches Syndrom und Sepsis

Das Kriterium einer Brandwundensepsis ist die Invasion der Mikroorganismen in tiefere Gewebsschichten der Haut, das Eindringen in perivaskuläre Strukturen, die Penetration der Gefäßwände und die Ausbreitung im Systemkreislauf mit den entsprechenden Folgen bis hin zum progressiven Multiorganversagen. Der Nachweis von Keimen in der Blutkultur trotz systemischer Ausbreitung bleibt oft negativ, so daß die Bewertung der Blutkultur nur im positiven Fall diagnostische Aussagen erlaubt. Die histologische Untersuchung und die quantitative Keimzahlbestimmung von Biopsieproben bieten sich als zusätzliche verlässlichere Parameter einer mikrobiellen Invasion an [42]. Das septische Syndrom ist durch klinische Symptome gegeben: u.a. Fieber, Kreislaufversagen, Hypermetabolismus, Verwirrungszustände oder eine Leukozytose, an die sich prämortal oftmals eine Leukopenie anschließt [6].

Die Synthese und Exkretion mikrobieller Toxine ist offensichtlich für die Kolonisierung, Invasion und Überwindung der körpereigenen Infektabwehr durch Mikroorganismen eine wesentliche Voraussetzung. Andererseits aktivieren z.B. die Lipopolysaccharide (Endotoxine) gramnegativer Bakterien auch das Immunsystem. Kennzeichen dafür ist die Induktion von Cytokinen (u.a. IL1, IL-6 oder TNF-α) oder Entzündungsmediatoren wie Leukotriene [7, 27].

Das Endotoxin gramnegativer Bakterien [40] ist prinzipiell nicht alleiniger Induktor der klinischen Sepsis-Symptome, die ja ebenfalls bei der Sepsis hervorgerufen durch grampositive Bakterien (z.B. beta-hämolysierende Streptokokken oder Staphylokokken) auftreten. Offensichtlich spielen neben den bisher gut untersuchten Endotoxinen eine Vielzahl anderer bakterieller Toxine und Pathogenitätsfaktoren bei der Ausprägung des septischen Syndroms eine Rolle.

Während die „Infektion" ein mikrobiell zugeordnetes Charakteristikum ist, reflektiert das „septische Syndrom" und die „Sepsis" eher die Antwort der körpereigenen Infektabwehr auf das Trauma und die mikrobielle Kolonisierung [6, 29].

Typischerweise kann das septische Syndrom experimentell auch ohne mikrobielle Pathogenitätsfaktoren z.B. durch Injektion von IL-1 oder TNF-α induziert werden. Träger des septischen Syndroms sind damit Cytokine und Entzündungsmediatoren [29]. Dennoch ist die physiologische Aufgabe dieser Mediatoren das Immunsystem zu aktivieren und zu kontrollieren. Für die Ausprägung der pathophysiologischen Symptomatik spielt dann das Zusammentreffen vieler Faktoren eine Rolle, zu denen u.a. die Überproduktion von Cytokinen über einen längeren Zeitraum gehört.

Überschießende Cytokin-Synthese: IL-6

Die pleiotropen Wirkungen des IL-6 erstrecken sich auf die Differenzierung von B-Zellen in antikörpersezernierende Plasmazellen, die Steigerung von T-Zellfunktionen (Proliferation, Cytotoxizität), und die Stimulation der Hämatopoese im Synergismus mit IL-3 [1]. IL-6 ist ein wichtiger Induktor der Akutphasenprotein-Synthese in der Leber und wirkt als endogenes Pyrogen. Es wird von einer Vielzahl von Zellen (z.B. Monozyten, Makrophagen, Endothelzellen, Fibroblasten, Lymphozyten) gebildet [1]. Klinische Untersuchungen zeigten eine Erhöhung der IL-6 Plasmakonzentrationen bei akuten bakteriellen Infektionen, in der Akutphase nach einem Verbrennungstrauma, bei Transplantationsabstoßungsreaktionen sowie bei entzündlichen Gelenkserkrankungen [14, 30, 32]. Wir konnten zeigen, daß auf der Regulationsebene der Cytokine das Interleukin 6 dramatisch im Plasma der Brandverletzten ansteigt [32].

Insbesondere bei dem Vergleich von Patienten mit unterschiedlichem klinischem Verlauf wurde das sehr deutlich. Bei überlebenden Patienten fällt der Plasma-IL-6-Spiegel nach initialem Anstieg. Im Gegensatz dazu stand der massive Anstieg von IL-6 besonders in der Spätphase bei verstorbenen Patienten, die zu diesen Zeitpunkten eine dokumentierte Sepsis durchliefen. Zusätzlich konnten wir auch die vermehrte in-vitro IL-6-Bildung von isolierten mononukleären Zellen Brandverletzter sowie den erhöhten Messenger-RNA-Gehalt dieser Zellen nachweisen [32].

Cytokine und lösliche Cytokin-Rezeptoren

Das systemische Ansteigen von bestimmten Cytokinen ist ein wesentliches Charakteristikum während der Sepsis und des septischen Schocks. Zu diesen Cytokinen gehören IL-1, IL-6, TNF-α oder TGFβ [11]. Zusätzlich ist die molekulare Struktur des erhöhten TNF bei Traumapatienten anders (27 kDa) als bei einem Normalspenderkollektiv. Das gilt sehr wohl für das Verbrennungstrauma aber nicht für alle Traumaformen. Bei experimentell-induzierter Hämorrhagie oder stumpfen Trauma fand man keine Erhöhung systemischer TNF-α-Spiegel [38].

Die biologische Aktivität der Cytokine ist häufig multifunktionell [1]. Dem TNF-α werden viele systemische und gewebsspezifische Schädigungen zugesprochen. Es gibt

Tabelle 1. Faktoren, die eine Cytokinwirkung beeinflussen

1. Cytokine können überschneidende Wirkprofile haben (z. B. IL-1 und TNF-α)
2. Cytokine können auf verschiedene Zellen wirken
3. Cytokine (z. B. TNF-α) induzieren Cytokine, d. h. eine Cytokinwirkung beruht evtl. nicht auf einem einzelnen Cytokin
4. Gleichzeitig anwesende Cytokine wirken synergistisch oder inhibitorisch
5. Cytokinrezeptoren auf den Zielzellen sind auf- oder abreguliert
6. Cytokine werden durch lösliche Cytokinrezeptoren neutralisiert (z. B. IL-2 oder TNF)
7. Cytokine interagieren mit anderen Mediatoren (z. B. Eicosanoiden oder Neuropeptiden)

aber ebenfalls Hinweise dafür, daß TNF-α induzierbare biochemische Reaktionen wie z.b. die Synthese von Stickoxid (NO) oder Lipid-Mediatoren für terminale Noxen verantwortlich sind. Die TNF-α-Produktion in Makrophagen von Trauma-Patienten ist insensitiv gegenüber einer Gegenregulation durch PGE_2. Offensichtlich versagen hier Regulationsmechanismen (z.b. getragen durch IL-2), die sonst einer überschießenden Cytokinsynthese entgegenwirken. IL-1 steigt schon frühzeitig während der Ausbildung des septischen Syndroms an und fungiert u.a. als Induktor anderer Cytokine wie TNF-α.

IL-6 und IL-8 sind durch IL-1 wie auch durch TNF-α zu induzieren und üben spezielle Funktionen aus, die z.T. auch überschneidend sind. Für die cytokingetragenen pathophysiologischen Auswirkungen müssen offensichtlich mehrere der o.g. Faktoren aufeinander treffen. Dementsprechend muß man die traumainduzierte Immunsuppression als Nettoresultat der komplex veränderten Signalgebung sehen, deren Auswirkungen sich dann auch an einzelnen Zellpopulationen zeigen lassen (Tabelle 1).

Untersuchungen unserer Arbeitsgruppe haben zentrale Elemente dieser Immunsupression bei der spezifischen (Lymphozytensystem) und unspezifischen Infektabwehr (Granulozytensystem) aufzeigen und biochemisch charakterisieren können (Tabelle 2).

Die Granulozytendysfunktion

Wir wiesen nach daß der typische chemotaktische Funktionsverlust der Granulozyten multifaktoriell bedingt ist. So ist die Freisetzung chemotaktisch aktiver Faktoren nach Stimulation von Patientengranulozyten vermindert [19–21]. Für das neben IL-8 potenteste, körpereigene Chemotaxin Leukotrien B_4 (LTB_4) wurde eine reduzierte Bildung nachgewiesen. Zudem ist die Metabolisierung des freigesetzten LTB_4 zu inaktiven Produkten erhöht [10]. Zusätzlich ist auch die LTB_4-Rezeptorexpression auf Patientengranulozyten vermindert [8]. Die auf diese Weise herabgesetzte Fähigkeit der Phagozyten, ein chemotaktisches Potential aufzubauen, geht einer invasiven bakteriellen Infektion voraus oder stellt eine begleitende Funktionsstörung dar [19]. Selbstverständlich wird die komplexe Symptomatik der Verbrennungskrankheit auch durch die Vielfalt anderer biologisch aktiver Mediatoren geprägt. Außer dem Leukotrien B_4 sind auch die spasmogenen und vasoaktiven Cysteinyl-Leukotriene (LTC_4, LTD_4, LTE_4) von Bedeutung. Die enzymatische Inaktivierung der Cysteinyl-Leukotriene im Plasma ist in der Frühphase nach Verbrennung vermindert. Der Thrombozytenaktivierende Faktor (PAF), zu dessen bio-

Tabelle 2. Auswahl an Veränderungen der zellulären und humoralen Elemente der spezifischen und unspezifischen Infektabwehr nach Verbrennungstrauma

Neutrophile Granulozyten	verminderte Chemotaxis
	eingeschränkte Bakterizidie
	verminderte Phagozytose
	initial erhöhte, dann verminderte Chemilumineszenz
	verminderte LTB_4-Generierung
	verstärkter LTB_4-Metabolismus
	verminderte LTB_4-Rezeptorexpression
	verminderte PAF-Metabolisierung
	verminderte Basalexpression von Adhäsionsmolekülen (CD11b)
	verstärkte Aufregulation von CD11b nach Stimulation
	verminderte Aktin-Polymerisierung
	erhöhte GTPase-Aktivität
	erhöhte HSP-Expression
Basophile Granulozyten	verminderte Histaminausschüttung
Thrombozyten	verminderte 12-HETE-Generierung
Monozyten/Makrophagen	verminderte Antigenpräsentation
	verstärkte IL-1-Produktion
	verstärkte PGE_2-Produktion
	verstärkte IL-6-Produktion
	verstärkte TNF-α-Produktion
T-Lymphozyten	verminderte T-Zell-Proliferation
	initial verstärkte, dann verminderte IL-2-Produktion
	verminderte Produktion von IL3, IFN-γ, IL-5
	vermehrte Expression nicht-funktionsfähiger IL-2-Rezeptoren
	vermehrte Freisetzung von löslichen IL-2-Rezeptoren (sIL2R)
	erniedrigtes $CD4^+/CD8^+$-Verhältnis
B-Lymphozyten	verstärkte bzw. verminderte B-Zell-Proliferation
	zeitabhängig erhöhte Ig-Synthese
	verminderte CD23-Expression
	verminderte sCD23-Freisetzung
Plasma/Serum	zeitabhängige Verminderung der Komplementkomponenten
	erhöhte Cytokinspiegel (IL-6, TNF-α, TGFβ)
	erhöhte Spiegel löslicher Cytokinrezeptoren (sIL2R, sTNF-RI und RII)
	erhöhte IL-1ra-Werte
	erhöhte Ig (zeitabhängig)

logischen Wirkqualitäten u.a. die eosinophile Chemotaxis, die Bronchokonstriktion, die Induktion einer bronchialen Hyperreagibilität sowie die Modulation lymphozytärer Funktionen zählen, wird von neutrophilen Granulozyten schwerverbrannter Patienten in vermindertem Maße synthetisiert und metabolisiert [35]. Somit werden Lipidmediatoren wie LTB_4 oder PAF im Rahmen des Verbrennungstraumas unterschiedlich metabolisiert.

Die verminderte zelluläre Reaktivität ließ sich auch an basophilen Granulozyten schwerverbrannter Patienten zeigen [4]. So führten Zellstimulationen mit anti-IgE oder dem Ca-Ionophor A23187 zu einer verminderten Freisetzung von Histamin bei unverändertem Histamingehalt der Zellen.

Diese Daten belegen, daß auch durch das Fehlen von Mediatoren wie z.B. von Lipidmediatoren oder von biogenen Aminen der geordnete Ablauf der Infektabwehr beeinträchtigt werden kann.

Neue Untersuchungen zeigen, daß bestimmte Cytokine wie IL-6 oder TNF-α im Verlauf der posttraumatischen Phase im peripheren Blut ansteigen. Eigene Untersuchungen haben ergeben, daß TNF (α und β) die Expression von LTB_4-Rezeptoren auf Granulozyten gesunder Spender vermindert. Darüberhinaus konnten wir nachweisen, daß auch bakterielle Endo- oder Exotoxine *in vitro* die zelluläre Reaktivität von normalen Granulozyten herabsetzen [5, 7]. Durch die Verwendung definierter Zellstimuli (z.B. fMLP, Rezeptoragonist; NaF, G-Protein-Aktivator; Kalzium-Ionophor, direkter Kalziumioneneinstrom) konnten wir die Ursachen der Granulozytendysfunktion auch in Veränderungen der membranbiochemischen Signaltransduktion lokalisieren (G-Proteine, Aktinpolymerisierung, Adhäsionsmoleküle wie CD11b [9].

Die Suppression der spezifischen Immunantwort

Die Zellen des Phagozytosesystems und die Zellen der spezifischen Immunantwort (Antigenerkennung, Antikörperbildung, cytotoxische Funktionen) stehen über Entzündungsmediatoren wie PGE_2, LTB_4 oder PAF bzw. über Cytokine wie IL-1, IL-6, TNF-α oder IL-8 in Verbindung und beeinflussen sich so gegenseitig. Wir haben das nach Trauma veränderte spezifische Immunsystem u.a. anhand von lymphozytenfunktionen analysiert [31–34].

Unsere Ergebnisse haben gezeigt, daß beim Brandverletzten keine Verschiebung im Verhältnis zirkulierender T-, B- und Null-Zellen gegenüber Normalspendern zu finden ist. Demgegenüber ist allerdings eine Abnahme von Helfer/Inducer-T-Zellen (also CD4-Zellen) gegenüber den Suppressor/cytotoxischen T-Zellen (also CD8-Zellen) typisch. Diese Verschiebung des CD4/CD8-Verhältnisses dokumentiert zwar den immunsupprimierten Status des Brandverletzten, gibt uns aber keine Informationen zu funktionellen Zelleistungen.

Deswegen untersuchten wir die Proliferationsleistung von T- und B-Lymphozyten nach Stimulation mit PHA, einem T-zellspezifischen Mitogen, oder SAC, einem polyklonalen B-Zellaktivator.

Bei schwerverbrannten Patienten kommt es zwischen der zweiten und fünften Woche nach Trauma zu einer ausgeprägten T-Zellsuppression, während die B-Zellproliferation in geringerem Maße betroffen ist. Die polyklonale Immunglobulinsynthese Schwerverbrannter nach Stimulation mit PWM (Pokeweed Mitogen) oder SAC (S. aureus Cowan I) ist ebenfalls zwischen der zweiten und fünften Woche nach Trauma supprimiert. Antikörper der Frühphase einer humoralen Immunantwort (IgM) wie auch der Spätphase (IgG) sind dabei in gleicher Weise betroffen.

Die Befunde zur Lymphozytenproliferation und zur Antikörpersynthese deuten darauf hin, daß bei Schwerbrandverletzten die Aktivierung von T- und B-Zellen gestört ist. Deswegen untersuchten wir die Expression und Regulation der Lymphozytenaktivierungsmarker CD25 und CD23. CD25 ist vornehmlich ein Marker für aktivierte T-Zellen und Bestandteil des Rezeptors für Interleukin 2. CD23 ist ein B-Zellaktivierungsmarker und fungiert u.a. als Rezeptor für B-Zellwachstumsfaktoren.

Bei Schwerbrandverletzten kommt es in der zweiten bis fünften Woche nach Trauma zu einer Verringerung der Interleukin-4-stimulierten CD23-Expression. Gleichzeitig ist die spontane und Interleukin-2-stimulierte CD25-Expression deutlich gesteigert.

Diese Befunde sprechen für eine intrinsische B-Zell-Funktionsstörung und ebenfalls für eine gestörte Regulation über das T-Zell-System. Wir wissen inzwischen, daß es sich bei vermehrt exprimierten CD25-Komponenten um nicht-funktionelle IL2-Rezeptoren handelt. Hier liegen offensichtlich Entkopplungen im Signaltransduktionssystem vor.

Nicht nur die verminderte Bildung von regulatorischen Faktoren im Immunsystem kann zur Fehlregulation beitragen, sondern auch vermehrt gebildete Komponenten.

Stress-Proteine

Es ist offensichtlich, daß der schwerverletzte Patient einer Vielzahl psychischer und biochemischer Stressfaktoren ausgesetzt ist. Eine intrazelluläre Stressantwort ist u.a. die Bildung sogenannter Stressproteine (heat-shock proteins, hsp). Stressproteine werden z.B. durch Hypoxie oder Infektionen induziert. Experimentell kann man die Bildung von Stressproteinen durch die hypertherme Behandlung der Zellen hervorrufen. Die genaue physiologische Rolle von Stressproteinen ist noch nicht vollständig geklärt. Durch ihre Beteiligung an essentiellen intrazellulären Prozessen wie z.B. Proteintransport oder Proteinfaltung haben sie offensichtlich protektive Funktionen. So sind bestimmte Stressproteine in der Lage, bereits denaturierte Enzyme wieder zu reaktivieren [37]. Unsere Untersuchungen haben gezeigt, daß sowohl bakterielle Toxine als auch Cytokine (IL-6, TNF-α) und Lipidmediatoren (12-HETE) in der Lage sind, in peripheren Leukozyten Stressproteine zu induzieren [17, 23–25]. Diese Ergebnisse lassen einen Zusammenhang zwischen der intrazellulären Stressreaktion und der veränderten zellulären Reaktivität vermuten [21, 22]. Möglicher-

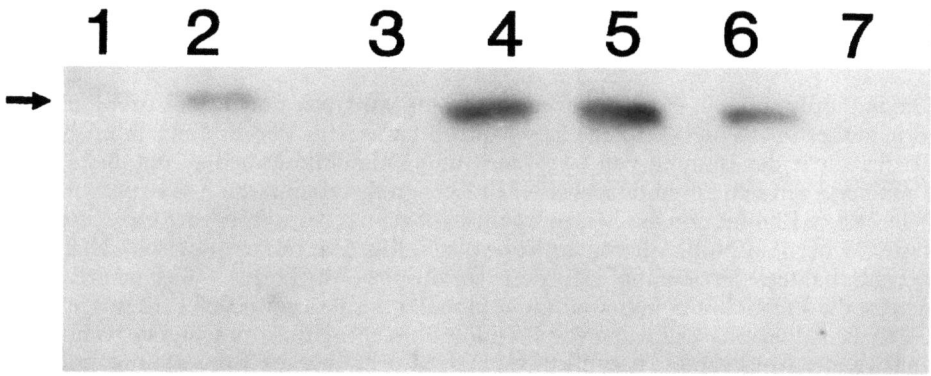

Abb. 1. Expression von Stress-Protein (hsp72; Pfeil) in humanen neutrophilen Granulozyten. 1: Normalspender A; 2: Normalspender B; 3–7: Patient mit manifester Sepsis. 3: Abnahmetag 1; 4: Abnahmetag 3, 5: Abnahmetag 7; 6: Abnahmetag 11; 7: Abnahmetag 20. Der Patient verstarb an sepsis-induziertem Multiorganversagen

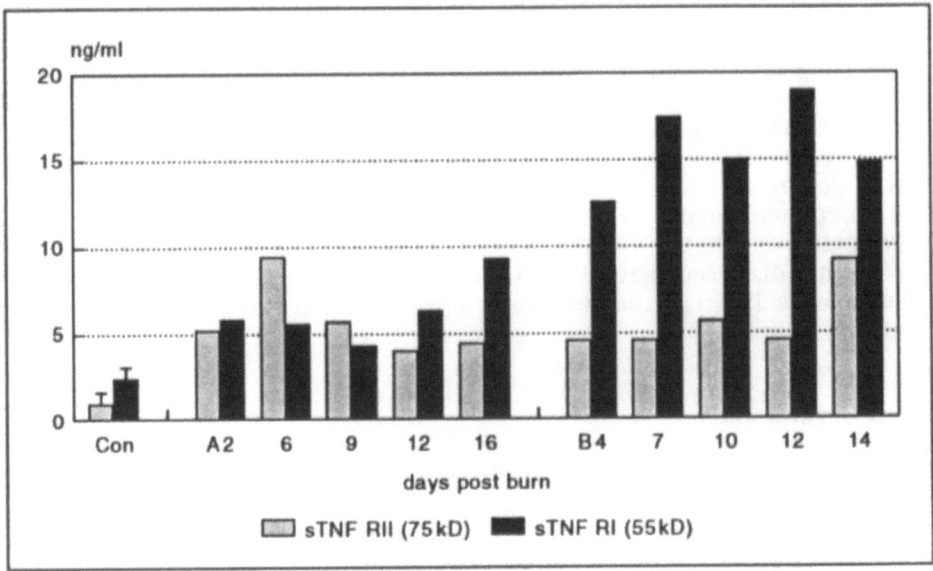

Abb. 2. Messung des TNF-Inhibitor (TNF-INH) als löslicher TNF-Rezeptor Typ I (sTNF-RI) und Typ II (sTNF-RII). Die Messung erfolgte durch Dr. Roux-Lombard, Genf. Con: Normalspender-Serum; A: Verbrennungspatient, weibl., 40 J., 48% verbrannte Körperoberfläche zweit- und drittgradig, zusätzliches Inhalationstrauma. B: Verbrennungspatient, männl., 49 J., 75% verbrannte Körperoberfläche zweit- und drittgradig, ab Tag 7 nV septisches Syndrom

weise reflektiert die Induktion von Stressproteinen einen intrazellulären Schutzmechanismus gegen bakterielle Toxine oder eine überschießende Cytokinexposition. Wie die Abb. 1 zeigt, konnten wir die Induktion von Stressproteinen (hsp72) in den peripheren Leukozyten eines Patienten mit manifester Sepsis nachweisen.

Therapeutische Ansätze

Die Pathophysiologie des septischen Syndroms wird von mindestens drei Parametern mitbestimmt: der Virulenz der Mikroorganismen, der Bildung mikrobieller Toxine sowie der Bildung von Cytokinen und Entzündungsmediatoren [6, 11, 29]. Damit ergeben sich auf unterschiedlichen Ebenen therapeutische Ansatzpunkte (Tabelle 3). Die Elimination der Mikroorganismen gelingt trotz moderner topischer und systemischer Antibiotikatherapie nicht vollständig. Die immunologische Neutralisierung bakterieller Toxine erfordert spezifische Antikörper. Vielversprechend scheint die Entwicklung humaner monoklonaler Antikörper gegen Endotoxin oder gegen die Adhäsionsstrukturen von Pseudomonas aeruginosa zu sein. Die rechtzeitig angewandte Antikörper-Therapie bietet in der Frühphase der Entwicklung und Verselbstständigung des septischen Syndroms die Möglichkeit einer frühen Maßnahme.

Wesentlich komplexer stellt sich die therapeutische Regulation der cytokin- und mediator-induzierten Symptomatik dar [15]. Hier ist es z.B. das Ziel, selektiv überschießende Cytokinproduktionen zu drosseln und gleichzeitig physiologische Cyto-

Tabelle 3. Mögliche zukünftige Therapiekonzepte

Toxinneutralisierung mittels monoklonaler Antikörper (z. B. anti-Endotoxin-Antikörper)
Cytokinneutralisierung mittels monoklonaler Antikörper (z. B. anti-IL-6 oder anti-TNF-α) oder lösliche Cytokinrezeptoren
Cytokin-Rezeptor-Blockade mittels monoklonaler Antikörper oder Rezeptor-Antagonisten (z. B. IL-1ra)
Cytokin-Kombinations-Therapie bzw. Cytokin-Peptid-Theapie zur Induktion erwünschter Cytokineffekte (z. B. Immunstimulation)
Reaktivierung „paralysierter" Zellfunktionen durch hämatopoetische Wachstumsfaktoren (z. B. G-CSF, GM-CSF), Interleukinen (z. B. IL-8) oder stabilen Eicosanoiden (z. B. LTB4-Agonisten)

---

kinspiegel zu erhalten, die eine geordnete Infektabwehr erst ermöglichen. Damit ist die pharmakologische Gesamtblockade einer Mediatorsynthese z.B. über Glucocorticoide oder Cyclosporin wenig sinnvoll, da eine bestehende Immunsuppression weiter verstärkt wird. Eher bieten sich Faktoren an, mit denen das Immunsystem selbst die Cytokinwirkungen steuert wie z.b. die natürlich vorkommenden Inhibitoren von IL-1 nämlich das TNF-α-Bindeprotein (TNF-INH) [12, 13]. IL-1ra ist dem IL1 strukturverwand, bindet an den IL1-Rezeptor, führt aber nicht zum Auslösen einer biologischen Antwort. TNF-INH ist ein lösliches Fragment des TNF-Rezeptors, bindet TNF-α und blockiert damit die Bindung von TNF an seinen Rezeptor. Wie wir nachweisen konnten, steigt TNF-INH als löslicher TNF-Rezeptor Typ I (TNF-RI) und Typ II (TNF-RII) mit jeweils unterschiedlichem Molekulargewicht nach Verbrennungstrauma im Plasma der Patienten stark an (s. Abb. 2).

Mögliche zukünftige Therapiestrategien sind in Tabelle 3 zusammengefaßt. Diese möglichen Therapiekonzepte lassen sich nur in interdisziplinärer Zusammenarbeit zwischen Klinik und Grundlagenforschung verwirklichen.

Abkürzungen:
CD, cluster of differentiation; G(M)-CSF, Granulozyten-(Makrophagen)-Kolonie-stimulierender Faktor; HETE, Hydroxyeicosatetraensäure; IFN, Interferon; Ig, Immunglobulin; IL, Interleukin; LT, Leukotrien; nV, nach Verbrennung; PG, Prostaglandin; TNF, Tumor-Nekrose-Faktor, TNF-INH, TNF-Inhibitor; sTNF-R, löslicher TNF-Rezeptor.

Literatur

1. Akira S, Hirnao T, Taga T, Kishimoto T (1990) Biology of multifunctional cytokines: IL6 and related molecules (IL 1 and TNF). FASEB J 4:2860–2867
2. Alexander JW, Gianotti L, Pyles T, Carell MA, Babcock GF (1991) Distribution and survival of Escherichia coli translocating from the intestine after thermal injury. Ann Surg 213:558–567
3. Arturson G (1985) Neutrophil granulocyte functions in severely burned patients. Burns 11:309–319
4. Bergmann U, König W, Gross-Weege W., Schlüter B, Köller M, Erbs G, Müller FE (1990) Basophil releasability in severely burned patients. J Trauma 30:1372–1379
5. Bergmann U, Scheffer J, Köller M, Schönfeld W, Erbs G, Müller FE (1989) Induction of inflammatory mediators (histamine, leukotrienes) from various cells by Pseudomonas aeruginosa strains from burn patients. Infect Immun 57:2187–2195
6. Bone RC, Fisher CJ, Clemmer TP, Slotman GJ, Metz CA, Balk RA (1989) Sepsis syndrome: a valid clinical entity. Crit Care Med 17:389–393

7. Bremm KD, König W, Thelestam M, Alouf JE (1987) Modulation of granulocyte functions by bacterial exotoxin and endotoxins. Immunology 62:363–371
8. Brom J, Köller M, Schönfeld W, Knöller J, Erbs G, Müller FE, König W (1988) Decreased expression of leukotriene B4 receptor sites on polymorphonuclear granulocytes of severely burned patients. Prostaglandins, Leukotrienes, Ess Fatty Acids 34:153–159
9. Brom J, König W, Brom C, Köller M, Hinsch KD, Spicher K, Erbs G, Müller FE Signal transduction in neutrophils of severely burned patients – Involvement of guanine nucleotide binding proteins. J Trauma, submitted
10. Brom J, König W, Köller M, Gross-Weege W, Erbs G, Müller FE (1987) Metabolism of leukotriene B4 by polymorphonuclear granulocytes of severely burned patients. Prostaglandins Leukotrienes Med 27:209–225
11. Cerra FB (1991) The systemic septic response: concepts of pathogenesis. J Trauma 30:S169–S174
12. Dayer JM (1991) Natural Inhibitors of interleukin-1 and tumor necrosis factor. In: Baxter A, Ross R (eds) Cytokine Interactions and their control. John Wiley & Sons Ltd., pp 51–57
13. Engelberts I, Stephens S, Francot GJM, van der Linden CJ, Buurman WA (1991) Evidence for different effects of soluble TNF-receptors on various TNF measurements in human biological fluids. Lancet 338:515–516
14. Guo Y, Dickerson C, Chrest FJ, Adler WH, Munster AM, Winchurch RA (1990) Increased levels of circulating interleukin 6 in burn patients. Clin. Immunol. Immunopathol 54:361–368
15. Haworth C, Feldmann M (1991) Applications of cytokines in human immunotherapy. In: The cytokine handbook. Academic Press, New York, pp 301–324
16. Hasslen SR, Nelsom RD, Kishimoto TK, Warren WE, Ahrenholz DH, Solem LD (1991) Down-regulation of homing receptors: a mechanism for impaired recruitment of human phagocytes in sepsis. J Trauma 31:645–652
17. Hensler T, Köller M, Alouf JE, König W (1991) Bacterial toxins induce heat shock proteins in human neutrophils. Biochem Biophys Res Commun 179:872–879
18. Jones WG, Minei JP, Barber AE, Fahey TJ, Shires GT (1991) Splanchnic vasoconstriction and bacterial translocation after thermal injury. Am J Physiol 261:H1190–H1196
19. Köller M, König W, Brom J, Raulf M, Gross-Weege W, Erbs G, Müller FE (1988) Generation of leukotrienes from human polymorphonuclear granulocytes of severely burned patients. J Trauma 28:733–740
20. Köller M, König W, Brom J, Schönfeld W, Erbs G, Müller FE (1989) Studies on the release of lipoxygenase products from granulocytes of severely burned patients. In: Faist E, Ninnemann J, Green D (eds) Immune Consequences of Trauma, Shock and Sepsis. Springer-Verlag, Berlin Heidelberg New York, pp 252–257
21. Köller M, König W, Brom J, Erbs G, Müller FE (1989) Studies on the mechanisms of granulocyte dysfunctions in severely burned patients – evidence for altered leukotriene generation. J Trauma 29:435–444
22. Köller M, Puchtler C, Brom J, König W. (1989) Inhibition of leukotriene generation from human polymorphonuclear granulocytes after heat-shock treatment. Prostaglandins Leukotrienes Ess. Fatty Acids 38:99–106
23. Köller M, Brom C, König W (1990) The influence of heat shock treatment on functional activities of human granulocytes, monocytes and platelets. In: Burdon R, Rice-Evans C, Blake D, Winrow V (eds) Heat Shock Proteins in Inflammation, Richelieu Press, London, pp 337–360
24. Köller M, König W (1990) Arachidonic acid metabolism in heat shock treated human leukocytes. Immunology 70:458–464
25. Köller M, König W (1991) 12-Hydroxyeicosatetraenoic acid (12-HETE) induces heat shock proteins in human leukocytes. Biochem. Biophys. Res Commun. 175, 804–809
26. Krüger C, Schütt C, Obertacke U, Joka T, Müller FE, Knöller J, Köller M, König W, Schönfeld W (1991) Serum CD14 levels in polytraumatized and severely burned patients. Clin Exp Immunol 85:297–301
27. Lehmann V, Freudenberg MA, Galanos C. (1987) Lethal toxicity of lipopolysaccharide and tumor necrosis factor in normal and D-gàlactosamine-treated mice. J Exp Med 165:657–663
28. Luterman A, Dasco CC, Curreri PW (1986) Infections in burn patients. Am J Med 81 (Suppl.):45–52

29. Marshall J, Sweeney D (1990) Microbial infection and the septic response in critical surgical illness. Arch Surg 125:17–23
30. Nijsten MW, Hack CE, Helle M, ten Duis HJ, Klasen HJ, Aarden LA (1991) Interleukin-6 and its relation to the humoral immune response and clinical parameters in burned patients. Surgery 109:761–767
31. Schlüter B, König W (1990) Microbial pathogenicity and host defense mechanisms- crucial parameters of posttraumatic infections. Thorac. Cardiovasc Surgeon 38:339–347
32. Schlüter B, König B, Bergmann U, Müller FE, König W (1991) Interleukin 6: a potential mediator of lethal sepsis after major thermal trauma: evidence for increased IL-6 production by peripheral blood mononuclear cells. J Trauma 31:1663–1670.
33. Schlüter B, Köller M, König W, Erbs G, Müller FE (1989) Studies on B-lymphocyte dysfunction in severely burned patients. J Trauma 30:1380–1389
34. Schlüter B, König W, Köller M, Erbs G, Müller FE (1991) Differential regulation of T- and B-lymphocyte activation in severely burned patients. J Trauma 31:239–246
35. Schönfeld W, Kasimir S, Köller M, Erbs G, Müller FE, König W (190) Metabolism of platelet-activating-factor (PAF) and lyso-PAF in polymorphonuclear granulocytes from severely burned patients. J Trauma 30:1554–1561
36. Shires GT (1991) Evolution of trauma and trauma research. J Trauma 30:S107–S115
37. Skowyra D, Georgopoulos C, Zylicz M (1990) The E. coli dnak gene product, the hsp70 homolog, can reactivate heat-inactivated RNA polymerase in an ATP hydrolysis dependent manner. Cell 62:939–944
38. Stylianos S, Wakabayashi G, Gelfand JA, Harris BN (1991) Experimental hemorrhage and blunt trauma do not increase circulating tumor necrosis factor. J Trauma 31:1063–1067
39. Teodorczyk-Injeyan JA, Sparkes BG, Mills GB, Peters WJ (1991) Immunosuppression follows systemic T lymphocyte activation in the burned patient. Clin Exp Immunol 85:515–518
40. Ulevitch RJ, Mathison JC, Schumann RR, Tobias PS (1991) A new model of macrophage stimulation by bacterial lipopolysaccharide. J Trauma 30:S189–S192
41. Winkler M, Erbs G, Müller FE, König W (1987) Epidemiological studies on the microbial colonization in heavily burnt patients. Zbl Bakt Hyg, B 184:304–320
42. Winkler M, Erbs G, Müller FE, König W (1987) Comparison of methods for the quantitation of bacteria in burn wounds. Zbl Bakt Hyg, A 256:82–98
43. Winkler M, Erbs G, Müller FE, König W (1989) In vitro Virulenz wundinfizierender Staphylokokken-Isolate von schwerbrandverletzten Patienten. Langenbecks Arch Chir 374:181–184

Für die Verfasser:
Dr. rer. nat. M. Köller
Lehrstuhl für Medizinische Mikrobiologie und Immunologie,
Arbeitsgruppe Infektabwehrmechanismen
Ruhr-Universität Bochum
Universitätsstraße 150
D-44801 Bochum

The hypermetabolism of major thermal burn: Implications for infections

D. N. Herndon, T. C. Rutan, and D. Fleming

Shriners Burns Institute and University of Texas Medical Branch, Galveston, Texas, USA

The decade of the 1980s saw a tremendous diminution of mortality in major thermal burn injuries. Early massive excision and grafting of burns has increased the LD_{50} to 98% total body surface area (TBSA) burn in referral pediatric burn centers such as the Shriners Burns Institute-Galveston Unit. We believe that early excision of the burn wound, within 72 h of the time of injury, is absolutely essential in the very largest of 3rd degree burns, and we advocate, as a standard of care, the use of fresh cadaver skin as a temporary cover. We initially thought that excising and grafting the acute burn wound would return the patients' immunologic and hypermetabolic responses to normal. Surprisingly, this has not been the case; the physiologic and metabolic alterations following thermal injury continue despite these measures. Essentially, a burn patient is one whose outer defense, the skin, is breached and whose inner defense mechanism is deranged.

The major actor in postburn immunosuppression appears to be the macrophage/monocyte which modulates helper/suppressor T-lymphocyte ratios and natural killer cell (NK) levels. The macrophage also synthesizes complement, generates plasminogen, and contributes to the microvascular clots that lead to the increased microvascular permeability near the burn wound and in other organs. The macrophage, activated in the burn wound and in the lungs, releases chemoattractants that cause neutrophil migration and margination, in turn causing increased vascular permeability which is particularly troublesome in the smoke-injured lung. Production of vasoactive substances, such as thromboxane (TxB) and leukotrienes, is a recurrent theme following burn injury, and may augment the extent of the injury. The macrophage, in addition to recruiting leukocytes, also releases substances that modulate burn wound healing, alter immune function, and up-regulate metabolism. We believe that the hypermetabolic response to trauma is primarily mediated by the macrophage.

In no other disease or trauma state is the hypermetabolic response as great as it is in burn-injury. Patients with multiple fractures, peritonitis, and cancer have shown fractional increase in metabolic rate [1, 2], but massive burn injury can drive metabolic rate to twice normal. Generally, this hypermetabolic response can be blunted to 40–60% above normal, if the patient is wrapped in bulky dressings and kept warm with external radiant heating devices. The postburn response is also characterized by an increase in heart rate, with rates of 180–200 beats per minute (bpm) being common for children. A true upward central temperature reset occurs between the 5th and 15th post burn day and remains elevated for up to 2 months in injuries of greater than 60% total body surface area, regardless of the timing of burn wound closure. The temperature reset results in a core temperature that is around 38.6 °C [3, 4]. If we try to decrease core temperature, by cooling or by use of antipyretics, patients produce more heat to compensate.

We maintain or increase body heat on a cellular level by cycling glucose to phosphate and back, fructose to fructose-1-phosphate and back, and fatty acids and glycerol to triglycerides and back. These are all normal futile cycles that occur to produce energy and heat. Recent investigations have led us to understand that this is a catecholamine-influenced substrate cycling that maintains body temperature 2°C above normal [5, 6]. The metabolic expenditure of burn injury can be decreased by warming the environment to about 32–34°C. For the burned patient, thermal neutral is 33°C, the temperature at which they are most comfortable. Whether elevated core temperature is good or bad is a philosophical point. We believe temperature elevation through substrate cycling allows a more sensitive hormonal control on a cellular basis, so we hypothesize that increased temperature is appropriate in these patients. We do know that our current attempts to decrease temperature are counterproductive.

The afferent stimulus that causes this hypothalamic temperature reset, we believe, are monokines and prostanoids, specifically thromboxane, released from the inflammatory burn wound. Catecholamine levels are elevated six-fold and glucose flow is elevated three- to six-fold in burn patients relative to normal controls. Also increased are glucagon and cortisol, while insulin is near normal. However, the ratio of the catabolic hormones (catecholamine and glucagon) to insulin is markedly elevated. Whether we feed burn patients or not, peripheral protein is catabolized, resulting in a net negative nitrogen balance.

Although we deliver sufficient enteral calories to maintain total body weight, total body composition changes. Weight is distributed more to fat than to lean body mass. Patients catabolize protein and become peripherally spindly and centrally fat. Their livers become grossly enlarged as the Kupffer cells are engorged with fat. All this contributes to the burn patient's eventual morbidity. The macrophage establishes a hormonal milieu that is not significantly altered by either early surgery or by aggressive feeding.

In the rat model, we have been able to decrease the hypermetabolism post burn by adrenalectomy either with or without steroid support [4]. Thus, the adrenal medulla, or epinephrine, is a primary mediator of the hypermetabolic response. In humans, one would expect that beta adrenergic blockade would decrease the hypermetabolic response. We demonstrated that intravenous propranolol (1 mg/kg every 6 h) effectively decreased heart rate in children with major burns to a more effective range for cardiac pumping activity [7]. The patients became relaxed, left-ventricular stroke work index improved, and myocardial oxygen consumption decreased. However, propranolol did not affect resting energy expenditure. As we gave the beta blocking agent, glucagon levels increased in a reciprocal fashion.

In burned humans, elevated catecholamines, glucagon and glucocorticoids conspire to break down protein from skeletal muscle peripherally and recycle it to the liver where gluconeogenesis occurs. We thought that supplying new glucose, in the form of total parenteral nutrition (TPN), would decrease morbidity and mortality in these patients. Actually, TPN, starting at day 1 post burn, increased morbidity and had a great negative impact on the immune system in a large series of patients [8, 9]. We now recommend that TPN be used only when the enteral route is incapacitated. Almost all burn patients, even those over 80–90% TBSA, can be supported with continuous enteral feedings to provide adequate amounts of calories.

In burns of 60% TBSA 10 days post injury, leukocyte function is dramatically reduced [10]. Although the white cell counts are elevated to normal, leukocyte ability to phagocytize bacteria and to consume oxygen, an index of their ability to kill bacteria, is less than controls. This is not a plasma-mediated event; the cells are either immature or old and fatigued and they do not work well at all. T-cell phymotic markers show similar ravages that we think are primarily due to this conspiracy of signals. In a series of large burns with controls of the same age, the OKT3s are decreased significantly in burn patients relative to controls [11]. Again the helper/suppressor cell ratio is reversed from what one considers as reasonable.

A massive burn injury produces tremendous amounts of antigen. We believe the macrophage is releasing messengers in an attempt to prevent an accidental autoimmune response as seen in certain other disease conditions. Not only are the T-cell helper/suppressor ratios reversed, but responses to phytohemagglutinin (PHA) are markedly depressed up to 14 days post injury in rat burn models and up to 60–70 days post injury in humans. The most disturbing cellular defect, and the one that has been predictive of mortality, has been a defect in NK cells [12].

NK cells have Fc receptors for IgG and are functionally important in immunosurveillance against tumors and viral infection. Animal studies show that high NK activity causes an increased resistance to viral infections [13]. Unfortunately, almost all of our patients convert to positive for CMV and HSV. Natural killers suppress both B and T cell responses in states such as Kawasaki syndrome, Crohn's disease, multiple sclerosis, chronic lymphocytic leukemia in children syndrome and in major burn injury [14, 15]. Natural killer cells are extremely defective after major burn injury and are more defective in patients who die than in those who live [12]. Of those who die, all die with viral manifestations.

In large burns, the percent NK activity in nonsurviving patients studied at the height of the hypermetabolic response was quite low [12]. This defect in NK activity can be identified almost immediately post burn, which allows some prediction of survival. This defect gradually returns to normal as the patient recovers.

The suppressive activity of burn serum can be expressed on normal NK cells [16]. This is a serum-dependent phenomenon in contrast to the leukocyte abnormality discussed before. In this circumstance, NK cells from normal controls incubated with burn serum will be depressed. This depression is heat sensitive and not removed by dialysis.

We have tried some "magic bullets" to improve postburn immune response. Isoprinosine, a salt of paracetaminobenzene, enhanced blastogenic response of peripheral blood to PHA and concanavalin A (Con A) [17]. In a murine model, isoprinosine, in high concentrations, inhibited induction of suppressor cells by Con A and restored the antigen presenting capabilities of autoimmune responses. A similar improvement in our animal model was seen when interleukin 2 (IL-2) was used [18]. IL-2 is one of few naturally occurring immunostimulators and it also appears to decrease the hypermetabolic response. It appeared effective over a wide dosage range.

The condition most commonly associated with mortality following thermal injury is inhalation injury [19], and the leukocyte plays a major role. Twenty to 84% of all burn deaths are associated with smoke-inhalation injury [20]. In our experience, a large burn (>50% TBSA) with significant inhalation injury is uniformly fatal in adult patients. Inhalatation injury is a dramatic display of the immune response gone awry. We have found that white blood cells are primarily responsible for much of the pulmonary damage following inhalation injury. It is the leukocyte and its release of proteolytic enzymes and free oxygen radicals that kills burn patients.

As cells are destroyed and pulmonary alveolar macrophages are stimulated by the injury, chemotactic factors are released which bring leukocytes into the lung in large numbers. The injury is actually worsened due to the body's response to the injury. Polymorphonuclear leukocytes (PMNs) marginate in the pulmonary vasculature and migrate into the parenchyma [20], where they are activated and release proteolytic enzymes, free oxygen radicals and eicosanoids. Enzymes and free radicals destroy mucosa and cause pulmonary vascular hyperpermeability. Eicosanoids, such as thromboxanes and prostacycline, alter blood flow and pulmonary vascular pressures. Interstitial pulmonary edema develops and is followed by fluid leaking into the tracheobronchial tree and alveoli. Intra-alveolar edema and hemorrhages occur along with damage to type-I pneumocytes. Exposure of the alveolar basement membrane leads to hyaline membrane formation and further cast formation, resulting in inadequate alveolar oxygen exchange. All of these factors (noncardiogenic pulmonary edema, decreased lung compliance, increased pulmonary transvascular protein flux, hyaline membrane formation and shunting of blood in the pulmonary vasculature) contribute to the respiratory failure following inhalation injury. The damaged tracheobronchial epithelial surface and lung parenchyma are easy targets for opportunistic infections. Gut flora and pathogens from the infected burn wound (*Staph*, *E. coli* and *Pseudomonas*) are the most frequent organisms associated with the pneumonia developing after inhalation injury. If the patient does survive these insults, he is often left with significant lung disease from fibrosis and loss of alveoli associated with the disease process and its treatment.

Animal studies have demonstrated that if white blood cells, specifically PMNs, are depleted by nitrogen mustard or specific antibodies, most of the pulmonary damage following inhalation injury is blocked [21]. Extravascular lung water (EVLW) and measured lung lymph flow, both indicators of the amount of interstitial pulmonary edema, are decreased and eicosanoid release is attenuated. The animals do not develop irreversible pulmonary insufficiency and their lungs do not show the histologic changes typical of inhalation injury [21]. Removing white cells from the circulation is effective, but obviously impractical in humans. We have since turned to the use of specific proteolytic inhibitors and free-radical scavengers to decreased pulmonary complications of inhalation injury. A difficulty exists in that we must titrate these regimens to decrease the host response to reduce injury, but not to the point that we render the patient incapable of responding to infection.

Clearly, a number of other cells and substances play a role in the modulation of the postburn leukocyte function. Histamines, serotonin, and kallikreins are important. The basal epithelial cell in the lung and in the burn wound may be an important source of thromboxane and other vasoactive mediators. Damaged epithelial cells, in the lung and in the skin, directly release chemotactic factors and prime the macrophage. The macrophage profusely releases chemotactic factors which prime neutrophils and cause them to come to the site of injury where they sludge and release free oxygen radicals and proteolytic enzymes. This causes the formation of the characteristic copious exudate on the burn wound and in the lung. It also causes bronchoconstriction and prostanoid activation which cause a hypermetabolic response protein degradation/bronchoconstriction in the lungs.

There is some mechanistic information to be gained from the use of all these agents. The early release of thromboxane causes pulmonary artery hypertension which can be reversed by the same antiprostanoids that decrease the metabolic ravages. In randomized, controlled studies, we plan to use ibuprofen and other nonsteroidal anti-inflammatory agents in burn patients to block thromboxane production. Hopefully, we will suppress the ravages of the deranged host response, but not depress the normal host immunocompetence. We think this is an exciting frontier of burn treatment.

References

1. Bancroft GJ, Shellam GR, Chalmer JE (1981) Genetic influences on the augmentation of natural killer cells during murine cytomegalovirus infection: correlation with patterns of resistance. J Immunol 126:988
2. Basadre JO, Sugi K, Traber LD, Niehaus GD, Herndon DN (1988) Effect of leukocyte depletion on smoke inhalation injury in sheep. Surg 104:208
3. Bender BS, Winchurch RA, Thupari JN, Proust JJ, Adler WH, Munster AM (1988) Depressed natural killer cell function in thermally injured adults: Successful *in vivo* and *in vitro* immunomodulation and the role of endotoxin. Clin Exp Immunol 71:120
4. Goodall MC, Stone C, Haynes BW Jr (1957) Urinary output of adrenaline in severe thermal burns. Ann Surg 145:479
5. Herndon DN, Wilmore DW, Mason AD Jr, Pruitt BA Jr (1978) Development and analysis of a small animal model simulating the human postburn hypermetabolic response. J Surg Res 25:394
6. Herndon DN, Thompson PB, Traber DL (1985) Pulmonary injury in burned patients. Crit Care Clin 1:79
7. Herndon DN, Stein MD, Rutan TC, Abston S, Linares H (1987) Failure of TPN supplementation to improve liver function, immunity, and mortality in thermally injured patients. J Trauma 27:195
8. Herndon DN, Barrow RE, Rutan TC, Minifee P, Jahoor F, Wolf RR (1988) Effect of propranolol administration on hemodynamic and metabolic responses of burned pediatric patients. Ann Surg 208:484
9. Herndon DN, Barrow RE, Stein M (1989) Increased mortality with intravenous supplemental feeding in severely burned patients. J Burn Care Rehabil 10:309
10. Kinney JM, Long CL, Gump FE, Duke JH Jr (1968) Tissue composition of weight loss in surgical patients: I. Elective operations. Ann Surg 168:459
11. Long CL, Spencer JL, Kinney JM, Geiger JW (1971) Carbohydrate metabolism in man: Effect of elective operations and major injury. J Appl Physiol 31:110
12. Moran K, Munster AM (1987) Alterations of host defense mechanisms in burned patients. Surg Clin North Am 67:47
13. Silverstein P, Dressler DP (1970) Effect of current therapy on burn mortality. Ann Surg 171:124
14. Singh H, Berg N, Herndon DN (1988) Augmentation of rat natural killer cell activity by interleukin-2 and interferon following thermal injury. Proc Am Burn Assoc 20:19
15. Singh H, Herndon DN (1989) Effect of isoprinosine on lymphocyte proliferation and natural killer cell activity following thermal injury. Immunopharmacol-Immunotoxicol 11:631
16. Stein MD, Gamble DN, Klimpel KD, Herndon DN, Klimpel GR (1984) Natural killer cell defects resulting from thermal injury. Cell Immunol 86:551
17. Stein MD, Herndon DN, Klimpel G (1985) Burn patient serum suppression of natural killer activity. Proc Am Burn Assoc 17:56
18. Steinhauer EH, Doyle AT, Reed J, Kadish AS (1982) Defective natural cytotoxicity in patients with cancer: normal number of effector cells but decreased recycling capacity in patients with advance disease. J Immunol 129:2255
19. Wilmore DW, Long JM, Skreen RW, Mason AD Jr, Johnson DW, Pruitt BA Jr (1973) Studies of the effect of variations of temperature and humidity on energy demands of the burned soldier in a controlled metabolic room. Ft Sam Houston, US Army Institute of Surgical Research, Annual Report, Report Control Symbol MEDDH-288 (R1)
20. Wilmore DW, Long JM, Mason AD Jr, Skreen RW, Pruitt BA Jr (1974) Catecholamines: Mediator of the hypermetabolic response to thermal injury. Ann Surg 180:653
21. Ziegler HW, Kay NE, Zarling JM (1980) Deficiency of natural killer cell activity in patients with chronic lymphocytic leukemia. Int J Cancer 27:321

Author's address:
David N. Herndon, MD, Shriners Burns Institute, 815 Market St, Galveston, TX 77550

Ätiologie der Infektion, Infektionswege, Infektionskontrolle

Analyse des Keimspektrums und der Übertragungswege auf einer Verbrennungsintensivstation

D. Kistler, R. Jurek und R. Hettich

Klinik für Verbrennungs- und Plastische Wiederherstellungschirurgie
(Direktor: Prof. Dr. R. Hettich), Klinikum der RWTH Aachen

Die Zerstörung der Haut durch ein thermisches Trauma führt zu einem Verlust ihrer Schutzwirkung und einer Veränderung der Molekülarchitektur mit nachfolgender ausgeprägter Immunsuppression. Beide Faktoren begünstigen eine rasche und nahezu ungehinderte Bakterieninvasion über die Verbrennungsnekrose. Begünstigt durch die Mikrozirkulationsstörung in der Verbrennungswunde können weder körpereigene Abwehr noch potente Antibiotika an den Wirkungsort gelangen. Somit stellen die entstandenen Defekte einen idealen Nährboden für Keime dar.

Die an der Oberfläche unmittelbar nach dem Trauma keimarme oder gar sterile Wunde wird in der Regel rasch von Keimen der physiologischen Hautflora, zumeist wenig pathogene grampositive Kokken aus Haarfollikeln und Schweißdrüsen intakter Haut, besiedelt.

Nach einer gewissen Zeit werden die grampositiven Keime der ersten Phase zunehmend durch gramnegative Erreger verdrängt. Dieser Keimwechsel wird mit der größeren Neigung gramnegativer Bakterien zur Invasion und dem dadurch entstehenden Selektionsvorteil in Zusammenhang gebracht [20]. Diese Mikroorganismen stammen zu einem Teil aus dem Gastrointestinaltrakt des Patienten selbst, zum großen Teil aber aus seinem Umfeld, der Verbrennungsintensivstation. Dieses heterogene Erregerbild spiegelt das vielseitige Keimmuster des Patientenumfeldes wider, wobei die Keimspektren von Patient und Umfeld in einer gegenseitigen Wechselwirkung zueinander stehen [9, 12, 20]. Kontamination mit diesen Erregern bedeutet in vielen Fällen ein Überwuchern der ungefährlichen physiologischen Keime mit multiresistenten und aggressiven Mikroorganismen. Das Ziel jeder Behandlung muß folglich darauf ausgerichtet sein, durch geeignete Hygienemaßnahmen eine Übertragung gefährlicher Keime zu verhindern. Nur durch minutiöse Aufdeckung von Infektionswegen innerhalb einer Station und deren Unterbrechung ist eine Reduktion gefährlicher Keimbesiedlung möglich.

Material und Methoden

Die Untersuchungen wurden an 41 Patienten auf der Verbrennungsintensivstation unseres Klinikums vorgenommen. Das mittlere Alter aller Verbrennungspatienten betrug 39,5 Jahre (1–82 Jahre). Die mittlere Verbrennungsfläche der zweit- und drittgradigen Verbrennungen wurde auf 30,5 % der KOF (6–95 %) eingeschätzt. Die Verbrennungsopfer kamen unmittelbar von der Unfallstelle zur Aufnahme. Zu Beginn der Behandlung wurde bei allen Patienten ein Keimstatus durch Abstriche vom Haaransatz, den Achselhöhlen, der Anogenitalregion, den Extremitäten, aus dem Nasen-Rachen-Raum und den Verbrennungswunden erhoben. Anschließend erfolgte eine modifizierte Gerbungsbehandlung nach Grob. Gesicht und Hände wurden offen mit J-PVP oder mit J-PVP Gaze-Verbänden behandelt.

Nach der Primärbehandlung erfolgte die weitere Therapie auf der Verbrennungsintensivstation in Einheiten, die jeweils durch eine Schleuse von der übrigen Station abgetrennt sind. Patienten dieser Studie wurden ausschließlich in Einzelboxen behandelt. Vor Eintritt in die Behandlungszimmer wird die Schutzkleidung in der Schleuse gewechselt und eine Händedesinfektion durchgeführt. Vor Verlassen des Raumes wird die Kleidung erneut gewechselt und eine Händedesinfektion vorgenommen.

Zur Aufdeckung des Keimspektrums und der Infektionswege wurden die bakteriologischen Untersuchungen in 3 Bereiche unterteilt:

Untersuchung des Patienten: Zusätzlich zur bereits erwähnten Aufnahmeuntersuchung wurden tägliche Abstriche von den Verbrennungswunden bis zur völligen Abheilung der Defekte entnommen. Bei intubierten und beatmeten Patienten wurde routinemäßig im Abstand von 2 Tagen Trachealsekret zur Keimanalyse gewonnen. Beim Auftreten von Fieber oder Zeichen einer beginnenden Sepsis wurden je 2 arterielle und 2 venöse Blutkulturen angelegt sowie eine Urinprobe analysiert. Weiterhin wurden alle Katheterspitzen beim Wechsel oder nach Entfernung eingesandt.

Zur Klärung der Frage, ob es sich bei dem isolierten Keim um einen für den Patienten pathogenen Erreger handelt, wurde über die Entnahmeorte und den klinischen Zustand des Patienten zum Zeitpunkt der Entnahme genau Protokoll geführt und die Wundverhältnisse im Rahmen der Verbandswechsel dokumentiert.

Untersuchungen des Umfeldes: Hierbei ist das unmittelbare vom mittelbaren Umfeld des Patienten zu unterscheiden.

Zum unmittelbaren Untersuchungsgebiet gehören sämtliche potentielle Keimquellen in der nächsten Umgebung des Patienten. Für die Untersuchung wurden Abstriche und Abklatschpräparate von Bett, Waschbecken, Ablagen, medizinischen Geräten, Patientenkost, Griffen und Schaltern des Patientenzimmers entnommen.

Zum mittelbaren Untersuchungsgebiet rechnet man alle übrigen potentiellen Keimquellen, die räumlich vom Patientenzimmer getrennt sind, von denen jedoch eine indirekte Keimübertragung möglich ist. Für die Studie wurde Untersuchungsmaterial aus der Stationsküche (Waschbecken, Schwämme, Kühlschrank etc.), dem Akutlabor und der zentralen Überwachungseinheit gewonnen. Weitere Proben wurden von den gereinigten Betten und der Klimaanlage entnommen.

Die Untersuchung dieser Bereiche erfolgte durch unangekündigte Entnahmen im Abstand von 6–8 Wochen.

Untersuchung des Personals: Ebenfalls im Abstand von 6–8 Wochen wurden beim gesamten Personal Abstriche aus dem Nasen-Rachen-Raum entnommen. Zusätzlich gelangten Abstriche und Abklatschpräparate von Händen, Mundschutz, Kitteln und Schuhen zur Untersuchung.

Die Proben aus dem Umfeld und von der Personalkleidung wurden einer genauen Keimanalyse unterzogen. Zusätzlich wurde die Zahl der Kolonien bildenden Einheiten (KBE) angegeben. Hieraus ergibt sich eine gute Information über den momentanen Kontaminationsgrad der untersuchten Stelle.

Die aus den Abstrichen der Patienten angezüchteten Keime wurden bei 4 °C für einen längeren Zeitraum asserviert, um eine Vergleichsmöglichkeit mit später auftretenden Isolaten zu gewährleisten.

Zusätzlich erfolgte eine Phagotypisierung oder Bestimmung der Biovariante bei Staphylokokken und eine serologische Typisierung von Pseudomonas aeruginosa, um gleiche Stämme zu identifizieren. Damit wird die Voraussetzung geschaffen, eine Aussage über mögliche Kontaminationsquellen und -wege, wie auch über die Pathogenität eines Stammes zu erhalten.

Bei allen untersuchten Keimen wurden routinemäßig Antibiogramme erstellt, die beim Auftreten multiresistenter Keime auf zusätzliche, neuere Antibiotika erweitert wurden.

Für die Untersuchung wurden 793 Patienten- und Personalabstriche und 182 Umfeldproben ausgewertet.

Ergebnisse

Patientenabstriche: Die Analyse der Abstriche bei Aufnahme ergab in 56,6 % koagulasenegative Staphylokokken, bei 7,2 % Enterokokken und bei 36,2 % sonstige Keime. In 2 % fand sich eine Methizillinresistenz der koagulasenegativen Staphylokokken beim Aufnahmebefund, im Verlauf der Behandlung stieg diese auf 14 % an.

Aus Abbildung 1 kann entnommen werden, daß während des gesamten Beobachtungszeitraumes eine hohe Durchseuchung unseres Patientengutes sowohl mit koagulasenegativen Staphylokokken als auch mit St. aureus vorhanden war. Auffallend ist auch der große Anteil von Enterokokken bei den Wundinfektionen der Patienten. Die relativ große Zahl von Candida albicans ist Folge der teilweise sehr lange notwendigen Antibiotikatherapie.

Die Biotypisierung von 61 St. epidermidis bei insgesamt 31 Patienten während des Beobachtungszeitraumes ergab den Nachweis des gleichen Biotyps in 32 Fällen bei 14 Patienten. Dabei fand sich dieser Keim 25mal auf klinisch infizierten Wunden, 3mal auf unverletzter Haut, 1mal bei einem Vaginalabstrich und 3mal an einer ZVK-Spitze. Die weiteren 5 nachgewiesenen Biovarianten bei 29 Abstrichen dieses Keimes verteilten sich auf ingesamt 13 verschiedene Patienten. In 8 Fällen konnte dieser Keim als Sepsiserreger verantwortlich gemacht werden.

Ein ähnliches Bild ergab die Phagotypisierung des St. aureus. Es wurden 52 Keime von 17 Patienten typisiert. Auffallend war die Häufung zweier Biovarianten in 41 Fällen bei insgesamt 12 Patienten verteilt über den gesamten Beobachtungszeitraum. 35 Abstriche stammten von infizierten Wunden.

Bei 6,9 % der Patienten war Candida albicans nachweisbar, wovon 55 % von Wundabstrichen, 37 % aus dem Nasen-Rachen-Raum und der Trachea, sowie 5 % von Vaginalabstrichen stammten. Alle diese Patienten befanden sich wegen großflächiger Verbrennungen in einem schlechten Allgemeinzustand. Auf diesen Wunden fanden sich meist Mischinfektionen mit Proteus, E. coli, Citrobacter, Klebsiellen, koagulasenegativen Staphylokokken und Pseudomonaden.

Bei 12 von 37 Blutkulturen und 11 von 30 untersuchten Katheterspitzen bei Verdacht auf Septikämie gelang ein positiver Erregernachweis (=34 %). Wie aus Tabelle 2 ersichtlich, sind auch hier die koagulasenegativen Staphylokokken mit 71 % weit im Vordergrund. Selbst, wenn man ein Drittel als Folge möglicher Kontamination [6] abzieht, so verbleiben 47 %.

Bei der Serotypisierung von 38 isolierten Pseudomonaden fanden sich Typ A in einer Urinprobe, Typ J bei Wundabstrichen von 9 Patienten, Typ H bei 4 unterschiedlichen Umfeldproben sowie Typ E aus 8 Wundabstrichen eines Patienten, aus 10 Proben eines Patientenzimmers, in dem aber nicht der vorher genannte Patient lag und aus 7 Proben des Stationsumfeldes.

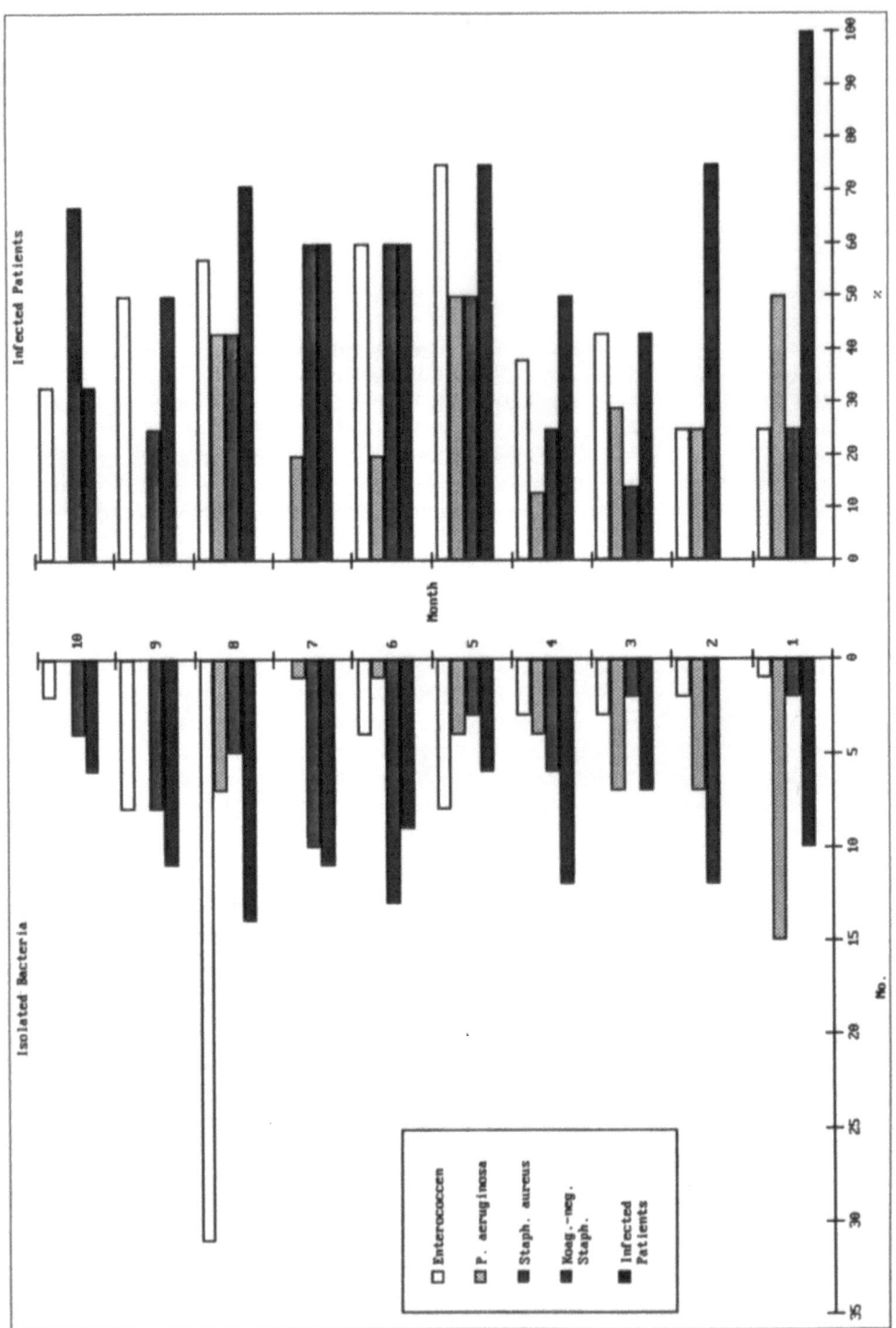

Tabelle 1. Veteilung der Keime bei den Patientenabstrichen

Koagulasenegative Staphylokokken	23,5%
Staphylococcus aureus	16,1%
Enterokokken	14,4%
Pseudomonas aeruginosa	12,6%
Candida albicans	6,9%
Proteus	5,9%
Streptokokken (außer D-Str.)	4,2%
Acetinobakter	4,0%
Enterobakter	3,76%
E. coli	2,5%
Serratia	2,2%
Klebsiella	1,4%
Übrige	2,5%

Tabelle 2. Verteilung der Keime bei positiven Blutkulturen und zentralen Kathetern

Staphylococcus epidermis	53%
Enterokokken	29%
Staphylococcus mitis	12%
Staphylococcus haemolyticus	6%
Pseudomonas aeruginosa	6%
Pseudomonas pichettii	6%

Anhand der Typisierung des Pseudomonas aeruginosa zeigte sich, daß bei einem Schwerbrandverletzten während des gesamten stationären Aufenthaltes derselbe Keim persistierte. Dieser Serotyp war mit drei unterschiedlichen Antibiotikaresistenzspektren aufgefallen. Zunächst fand sich nur die übliche Resistenz gegen SMZ-Trimethoprim. Im weiteren Verlauf, als sich der Patient in einem sehr schlechten Allgemeinzustand befand, traten dann zwei polyresistente Varianten auf. Gemeinsam war diesen die Resistenz gegen Azlocillin, Cefsulodin, Gentamicin, Tobramycin und Cefoperazon. Wegen der zu diesem Zeitpunkt nachgewiesenen schweren Mischinfektion erhielt er im Verlauf Piperacillin, Thienamycin bzw. Cefsulodin. Die Latenzzeit zwischen der ersten Gabe eines dieser Antibiotika und dem erneuten Nachweis desselben Serotypes betrug im Durchschnitt jeweils ca. 3 Tage. Die letzten bei dem Patienten nach Absetzen aller Antibiotika nachgewiesenen Pseudomonaden des gleichen Serotypes zeigten dann wieder das ursprüngliche Resistenzverhalten.

Umfelduntersuchung: Bei der ersten Umfelduntersuchung wurden bei 28 Proben 37 Keimkolonisationen nachgewiesen. In Tabelle 3 sind die relevanten Keime mit ihren Nachweisorten dargestellt.

Bei der nächsten Untersuchung wurden bei 31 Proben 36 Keimkolonisationen gefunden. In 14 Fällen fanden sich koagulasenegative Staphylokokken an der Arbeitskleidung, den Blutdruckmanschetten, sowie der Spüle und am Kühlschrank des Personalaufenthaltsraumes. In weiteren 6 Fällen zeigte sich St. aureus des gleichen

Abb. 1. Verteilung der 4 wichtigsten Keime während des Untersuchungszeitraumes links und gleichzeitig nachgewiesene Infektionen bei den Patienten durch die einzelnen Erreger rechts

Tabelle 3. Relevante Keimnachweise bei der ersten Umfelduntersuchung

Koagulasenegative Staphylokokken	Vernebler, Beatmungsgerät, Sondenkost, Stethoskop, Stauschlauch, Schutzkittel und OP-Hemd der Pflegekraft, Beatmungsbeutel, Bett, Anreichetisch
Enterokokken	Absauggerät, Sondenkost, Stethoskop, Salbendose, Schutzkittel der Pflegekraft
Proteus	Absauggerät (auch saubere Seite), Salbendose
Pseudomonas aeruginosa	Patientenbett
Klebsiella pneum.	Sondenkost
Enterobacter cloacae	steriles Abdecktuch des Anreichetisches

Tabelle 4. Verteilungsmuster der Keime aller Umfelduntersuchungen

Koagulasenegative Staphylokokken	36%
Anaerobe Sporenbildner	9%
Enterokokken	8%
Staphylococcus aureus	8%
Streptokokken (außer D-Str.)	6%
Pseudomonas	4%
Enterobacter cloacae	4%
Korynebakterium sp.	4%
Klebsiella	4%
Proteus	3%
Mikrokokken	7%
Gram (−) Bakterien	5%

Lysotyps bei mehreren Pflegekräften an der Schutzkleidung, den Schuhen, sowie am Mundschutz. Auch der Kühlschrankgriff war mit diesem Keim kontaminiert. Die auffallende Häufung dieses Keimes steht in einem direkten Zusammenhang mit der Infektion eines Kleinkindes mit dem selben Phagotyp.

Bei der nächsten unangemeldeten Umfelduntersuchung wurden 30 Proben mit 36 Keimkolonisationen gefunden. Auffallend war wieder der hohe Anteil koagulasenegativer Staphylokokken mit 17 Nachweisen an der Arbeitskleidung, den medizinischen Geräten, den Patientenkurven und der Zentrale. Bemerkenswert war das Auffinden von Pseudomonas aeruginosa aus einer Flasche mit phys. NaCl für die Zubereitung intravenöser Injektionen, aus der mehrfach entnommen werden kann. Die restlichen Nachweise setzten sich aus den unterschiedlichsten nicht relevanten Keimnachweisen zusammen.

Bei einer weiteren Untersuchung wurden nahezu identische Befunde erhoben.

In Tabelle 4 ist die prozentuale Verteilung aller bei den Umfelduntersuchungen nachgewiesenen Keime zusammengefaßt. Bemerkenswert ist auch hier der sehr hohe Anteil koagulasenegativer Staphylokokken, während die übrigen Erreger ein weitgehend gleichmäßiges Verteilungsmuster aufweisen.

Als interessanter Befund ergab sich der Nachweis von Enterokokken und St. aureus in einem vom Hersteller gewarteten und zur Wiederbenutzung bestimmten Luftbett. Diese Keime fanden sich auch später bei dem Patienten, der in diesem Spezialbett gelagert wurde.

Bei der Untersuchung der Filter der Klimaanlage konnte nur in einem Falle Pseudomonas aeruginosa nachgewiesen werden. Im gleichen Zimmer war bei acht aufgestellten Blutagarplatten nach 60minütiger Exposition und viertägigem Bebrüten nur eine KBE (Kolonie bildende Einheit) St. aureus darstellbar.

Personaluntersuchungen: Bei der Untersuchung der Abstriche vom Nasen-Rachen-Raum des Personals sind in wenigen Fällen koagulasenegative Staphylokokken nachgewiesen worden. Außerdem fanden sich St. aureus und jeweils einmal A-Streptokokken und Haemophilus influenzae. Insgeamt gesehen war die Anzahl der Keimträger beim Personal jedoch gering. Auffällig war allerdings die Häufung der Nachweise von St. aureus zu einem Zeitraum, in dem auch im Umfeld und insbesondere bei zwei Kleinkindern gehäuft der gleiche Lysotyp St. aureus nachgewiesen wurde, zu denen das Pflegepersonal einen engen Kontakt pflegte.

Die Untersuchung von Proben der Arbeitskleidung des Personals ergab nicht nur Kontamination der in der Schleuse zu wechselnden Schutzkittel mit pathogenen Keimen, sondern auch der ständig getragenen OP-Hemden und der darin befindlichen Utensilien wie z. B. Kugelschreiber.

Bei 7 Patienten fanden sich im Laufe der Behandlung Keime wieder, die bereits beim Aufnahmestatus nachweisbar waren. Bei 3 weiteren Patienten waren Wundinfektionen durch typische Keime der Darmflora aufgetreten.

Diskussion

Eine gute Übereinstimmung mit den Angaben aus der Literatur findet sich für die vier häufigsten Spezies, die alle mit über 10% an der Gesamtzahl der Abstriche beteiligt waren, nämlich koagulasenegative Staphylokokken, Staphylococcus aureus, Enterokokken und Pseudomonas aeruginosa, wobei die koagulasenegativen Staphylokokken jedoch eine Ausnahme bildeten [14, 22].

Diese Erreger galten bis Anfang der 80er Jahre in der Literatur als wenig pathogen. Der Nachweis der als physiologische Hautkeime bezeichneten Bakterien wurde als Kontamination und somit Abnahmefehler bezeichnet. Aus diesem Grunde wurde die Differenzierung dieser Keime vermutlich zu früh abgebrochen. In den letzten Jahren wurde jedoch zunehmend die Bedeutung der Staphylokokken bei der Auslösung schwerer Infektionen erkannt. So wurde auch über eine bedrohliche Zunahme von Septikämien durch koagulasenegative Staphylokokken berichtet [9, 19].

Die koagulasenegativen Staphylokokken waren in unserem Krankengut nach der Bewältigung gramnegativer Infektionen wieder gehäuft nachweisbar. Dieser Erreger war dann in erster Linie für Wundheilungsstörungen und St. aureus für die teilweise vollständige Zerstörung bereits eingeheilter Transplantate verantwortlich. Die Gefährlichkeit ergibt sich aber vor allem aus dem hohen Prozentsatz von 71% der positiven Blutkulturen bei unseren Patienten. Diese Ergebnisse stehen in gutem Einklang mit den Untersuchungen von Peters [19].

Die Verdrängung der Pseudomonaden als führender Keim bei Brandverletzten durch die Staphylokokken konnte bei unserem Krankengut bestätigt werden. Neu beschrieb noch 1983, daß bei 25% aller Verbrennungspatienten mit Pseudomonas Infektionen gerechnet werden muß [18]. Auch die Zahl von 97 Pseudomonas Nachweisen muß unter dem Gesichtspunkt korrigiert werden, daß 31 Nachweise von einem Patienten stammten, der über einen sehr langen Zeitraum mit diesem Keim behaftet war. Unsere Ergebnisse bestätigen eher die Beobachtungen von Mc Manus und Cross, die einen Rückgang der Pseudomonas Infektionen beschrieben [2, 16].

Als Grund ist wohl die gezieltere Verwendung der Antibiotika anzusehen, nachdem sich immer mehr die Kenntnis der Zusammenhänge zwischen prophylaktischer Antibiotikatherapie und Entstehung polyresistenter Keime durchsetzt. Gerade diese Gefahr scheint bei Pseudomonas aeruginosa besonders groß zu sein, wie die Serotypisierung der Isolate bei einem Patienten aufzeigen konnte. Ursache für die Ausbildung eines Pseudomonasstammes mit unterschiedlichen Resistenzen kann sowohl der Selektionsdruck der antimikrobiellen Therapie als auch die Begünstigung einer resistenten Unterart desselben Stammes aus einer heterogenen Infektionsdosis sein, wie dies von Krasilnikov gezeigt wurde [12]. Die Tatsache, daß vor allem Darmbakterien wie Escherichia coli und Enterobacter cloacae Resistenz-Plasmide auf P. aeruginosa und Klebsiellen übertragen können, veranschaulicht die Problematik der infektiösen Resistenz für die Therapie des Verbrennungspatienten [13]. Das ubiquitäre Auftreten und die rasche Änderung des Resistenzverhaltens bewirken die hohe Gefährdung für abwehrgeschwächte Patienten.

Die Verbrennungsintensivstation bildet ein Reservoir für die unterschiedlichsten Mikroben, die bereits mit einer großen Zahl Antibiotika in Berührung gekommen sind. Hierdurch haben sie zum Teil multiple Resistenzen entwickelt und persistieren für eine mehr oder wenig lange Zeit im Umfeld des Patienten. Durch direkten oder indirekten Kontakt mit den kontaminierten Gegenständen erfolgt schließlich eine Übertragung der Keime auf andere Patienten. Hierbei ist das Personal nicht so sehr Quelle der Infektion, als vielmehr mobiler Überträger in verschiedenen Infektionsketten [10]. Diese verlaufen direkt von Patient zu Patient, wenn beim Wechsel zu einem anderen Patienten keine neue Schutzkleidung angelegt und keine Händedesinfektion durchgeführt wird. Hambraeus und Laurell haben aufgezeigt, daß die Schutzkleidung des Personals, vor allem in Verbindung mit Nässe und Reibung, einen der Hauptinfektionswege auf der Verbrennungsintensivstation bedingt [10]. Durch die hohen Temperaturen in den einzelnen Behandlungsboxen kommt es aufgrund der Transpiration nach einiger Zeit zu einer vollständigen Durchnässung der gesamten Kleidung mit Übertritt der Keime, so daß auch das alleinige Wechseln des Schutzmantels beim Betreten des Patienzimmers nicht mehr ausreichend ist. Der große Anteil von nachgewiesenen Keimen auf der Kleidung des Personals unterstreicht die Notwendigkeit des mehrfachen Wechsels der gesamten Kleidung während einer Schicht. Wegen der großen Gefahr von Kreuzübertragungen ist anzustreben, daß während einer Schicht möglichst nur eine Schwester den Patienten betreut.

Nicht zu unterschätzen ist ferner die Infektionsgefahr durch kontaminierte Gegenstände im Patientenzimmer. Hier ist besonders darauf zu achten, daß bei Arbeiten am Patienten ständig Handschuhe getragen und diese häufig gewechselt werden.

Eine weitere sehr wichtige Kontaminationsquelle stellen die Gemeinschaftseinrichtungen der Intensivstation dar. Die Tatsache, daß gleiche Keime am Patienten ebenso wie im Umfeld auf der Station zu finden waren, zeigt, daß trotz Schleusen vor den einzelnen Patientenzimmern und vorgeschriebenem Wechsel der Schutzkleidung mit einer Händedesinfektion, eine beträchtliche Keimverschleppung innerhalb der Station erfolgte. Dies unterstreicht die Notwendigkeit der intensiven Unterweisung des Personals in die Hygienemaßnahmen und deren Einsicht. Da durch die hohe physische und psychische Belastung des Personals vereinzelt Nachlässigkeiten bei der Einhaltung der Hygienemaßnahmen nicht auszuschließen sind, sollten mindestens 2–3mal täglich Scheuerdesinfektionen der Gemeinschaftseinrichtungen erfolgen.

Wie schnell sich Hygienefehler auf die Verschmutzung der Station auswirken, zeigte insbesondere das Beispiel eines mit Staphylokokken infizierten Kleinkindes, welches aufgrund seiner sehr anhänglichen Art rasch die Zuneigung und den engen Kontakt zum Pflegepersonal gefunden hatte. Als Folge dessen waren nahezu sämtliche Gemeinschaftseinrichtungen nach kurzer Zeit mit dem Staphylokokkenstamm dieses Kindes kontaminiert.

Ein auch durch beste Infektionsprophylaxe nicht zu unterbindender Infektionsweg ist die Selbstkontamination des Verbrannten durch Translokation von Keimen aus dem Gastrointestinaltrakt. Diese kann bereits in den ersten Tagen nach der Verbrennung von großer Bedeutung sein [1, 8]. Durch einen frühzeitigen Beginn der enteralen Ernährung kann bei guter Darmfunktion dieser Mechanismus in vielen Fällen minimiert werden. Wegen der starken Beeinflussung der Darmflora durch orale Applikation von Antibiotika, sollte bei Verbrennungspatienten möglichst auf enterale Antibiotikagabe verzichtet werden. Inwieweit die hohe Infektionsrate der Patienten mit Enterokokken Folge einer Selbstkontamination oder mangelnder Hygiene ist, kann anhand der Daten kaum beantwortet werden. Auch ein Einfluß der routinemäßigen Ulkusprophylaxe ist hier möglich. Zunehmend gute Erfolge bei der Vermeidung von Translokation werden der selektiven Darmdekontamination zugeschrieben. Die Ergebnisse großer Studien sind allerdings noch abzuwarten.

Natürlich kann die unmittelbare Umgebung des Patienten niemals steril sein und es besteht auch keine große Gefahr für den Patienten, wenn es sich bei der Verschmutzung um seine eigenen Keime handelt. Es muß jedoch gesichert sein, daß die Keimzahl gering ist und eine weitere Ausbreitung verhindert wird. Bei unserer Untersuchung liegt aber der Schluß nahe, daß es sich am ehesten um Hygienefehler gehandelt haben könnte, wenn man die bei der Umfelduntersuchung festgestellte Kontamination der vom Pflegepersonal außerhalb des Patientenzimmers aufbereiteten Sondennahrung mit Enterokokken und Klebsiella pneumoniae kritisch betrachtet.

Die Auswertung der Abstriche aus dem Nasen-Rachen-Raum des Personals weist darauf hin, daß dieser für die Übertragung von Keimen nur eine untergeordnete Rolle spielt. Zu dem gleichen Schluß war auch Hambraeus in seiner Untersuchung gekommen [10]. Dieses Ergebnis gibt uns die Möglichkeit, die Vorschrift des ständigen Tragens des Mundschutzes zu lockern, was von den Patienten als sehr positiv empfunden wird. Allerdings muß einschränkend gefordert werden, daß bei längerdauernden Pflegemaßnahmen wie z.B. Verbandswechsel auch weiterhin Mundschutz getragen wird.

Der Keimstatus der Intensivstation bedarf einer ständigen Überwachung, um Schwachstellen möglichst rasch zu erkennen und geeignete Gegenmaßnahmen ergreifen zu können. Als Möglichkeit bieten sich in regelmäßigen Abständen von ein bis zwei Monaten unangekündige Umfelduntersuchungen an. Durch den Vergleich mit den bei den einzelnen Verbrennungspatienten isolierten Keimen sind die Infektionswege dann meist nachvollziehbar.

Literatur

1. Alexander JW, Gianotti L, Pyles T, Carey MA, Babcock GF (1991) Distribution and survival of Escherichia coli translocation from the intestine after thermal injury. Ann Surg 213: 558–567
2. Cross A (1983) Nosocomial infections due to Pseudomonas aeruginosa: Review of recent trends. Rev Infect Diseases, Suppl 5 (5):837–845
3. Curreri WP, Lutermann A, Braun DW, Shires GT (1980) Burn injury. Analysis of survival and hospitalisation time for 937 patients. Ann Surg 192:472–478
4. Daschner F, Langmaak H, Ahlborn B, Kümmel A (1983) Kontamination oder Sepsis. MMW 125 Nr. 39, 849–850

5. Deitch EA, Dobke M, Baxter CR (1985) Failure of local immunity. Arch Surg 120:78–84
6. Deitch EA, Maejima K, Berg R (1985) Effect of oral antibiotics and bacterial overgrowth on the translocation of the GI tract microflora in burned rats. J of Trauma 25 No. 5, 385–391
7. Deitch EA, Winterton J, Berg R (1986) Thermal injury promotes bacterial translocation from the gastrointestinal tract in mice with impaired T-cell-mediated immunity. Arch Surg 121:97–101
8. Desai MH, Herndon DN, Rutan RL, Abston S, Linares HA (1991) Ischemic intestinal complications in patients with burns. Surg Gynecol & Obstet 172:257–261
9. Fader RC, Hals PJ, Koo FCW (1987) Staphylococcal toxins: screening of burn wound isolates and evidence for alpha haemolysin production in the burn wound. Burns 13(6):462–468
10. Hambraeus A, Laurell G (1985) Verhütung von Wundinfektionen bei Verbrennungen unter besonderer Berücksichtigung der Schutzkleidung. Z gesamte Hyg 31 Heft 9, 508–511
11. Hettich R, Koslowski L (1984) Frühbehandlung der Brandwunden. Langenbecks Arch Chir 364:205–211
12. Krasilnikov AP, Adarchenko AA, Zmushko LS (1985) Sources of intrapopulation variability in causative agents of nosocomial infection. J Hyg Epidemiol Microbiol Immunol 29(2):169–176
13. Lowbury EJL (1979) Wits versus genes: The continuing battle against infection. J of Trauma 19 (1), 33–45
14. Maejima K, Deitch EA, Berg R (1984) Bacterial translocation from the GI-tract of rats receiving thermal injury. Infect Immun 43, No. 1:6–10
15. McManus AT, Mason AD Jr, McManus WF, Pruitt BA Jr (1985) Twenty five year review of Pseudomonas aeruginosa bacteremia in a burn center. Eur J Clin Microbiol April 219–223
16. McManus WF, Goodwin GP, Mason AD Jr, Pruitt BA Jr (1981) Burn wound infection. J Trauma 21:753–756
17. Mistry S, Mistry NP, Arora S, Antia NH (1986) Cellular immune response following thermal injury in human patients. Burns 12:318–324
18. Neu HC (1983) The role of Pseudomonas aeruginosa in infections. J Antimicr Chemoth Suppl B, 11:1–13
19. Peters G, Schumacher-Perdrau F, Pulverer G (1986) Infektionen durch Koagulase negative Staphylococcen bei abwehrgeschwächten Patienten. Immunität und Infektion Bd 14, 5:165–169
20. Peters G, Pulverer G (1984) Staphylokokken-bedingte Infektionen von implantierten Kunststoffmaterialien. Fortschr Antimikrob Antineoblast Chemother (FAC), Bd. 3–4, 469–474
21. Pruitt BA Jr, Colonel MC, McManus AT (1984) Opportunistic infections in severely burned patients. Am J Med March 30:146–154
22. Pruitt BA Jr, Lindberg RB (1979) Pseudomonas aeruginosa infections in burn patients. In: Dogett RG (ed) Pseudomonas aeruginosa. New York, Academic Press Inc., 339–366
23. Ransjö U (1986) Masks: a ward investigation and review of the literature. J Hosp Infect 7:289–294
24. Winkler M, Erbs G, Muller FE (1987) Epidemiologic studies of the microbial colonization of the burned patients. Zentralbl Bacteriol Microbiol Hyg [B] 184:304–320

Für die Verfasser:
Priv. Doz. Dr. D. Kistler
Klinik für Verbrennungs- und
Plastische Wiederherstellungschirurgie
der Medizinischen Fakultät der RWTH
Pauwelsstraße
D-52074 Aachen

Use of burn wound biopsies in the diagnosis and treatment of burn wound infection

B. A. Pruitt, Jr., A. T. McManus, S. H. Kim and W. G. Cioffi

US Army Institute of Surgical Research, Fort Sam Houston, USA

Improvements in both general care and wound care have favorably influenced the outcome of burn patients. Principal among these improvements have been the use of effective topical antimicrobial chemotherapy and the early postburn removal of ischemic nonviable burned tissue by excision, which have reduced the incidence of invasive burn wound infection as a cause of death [6]. Even so, current burn wound care is imperfect and certain patients, usually those with extensive burns that involve more than 50% of the total body surface (particularly children and the elderly), escape from microbial control and develop invasive burn wound infection [10].

The status of the burn wound must be monitored on a scheduled basis utilizing an integrated program of clinical, microbiologic, and pathologic examinations. The similarity of the systemic responses and the changes in laboratory values that accompany uncomplicated burn injury per se to those that accompany infection necessitates that reliance be placed on identifying changes in appearance of the wound that are produced by infections [9]. The wound must be examined at regularly scheduled (at least daily) intervals to identify changes in its appearance that are indicative of infection at a time when the process can be arrested and the patient salvaged.

The most frequent change in wound appearance due to invasive wound infection is focal, dark red, brown, or black discoloration of the eschar [12] (Table 1). Unfortunately, such color changes are nonspecific and can be caused by intraeschar hemorrhage due to minor local trauma. The most reliable sign of invasive burn wound infection is conversion of an area of partial-thickness injury to full-thickness skin necrosis. The alarming velocity with which those changes can occur is exemplified by the rapid centrifugal expansion of ischemic necrosis that is characteristic of invasive phycomycosis and the unexpectedly rapid separation of the eschar associated with fungal and yeast infections [7]. Unfortunately, such rapid eschar separation may also occur in the absence of invasive infection when the burn injury has been deep enough to cause liquifaction of the underlying subcutaneous fat. Certain clinical findings are characteristic of infections caused by specific microorganisms. Green discoloration of subcutaneous fat due to the metabolic product pyocyanin, and the presence of erythematous nodules that evolve into focal areas of eschar formation (ecthyma gangrenosum) are typical of pseudomonas infections. Violaceous discoloration of edematous unburned skin at the margins of the burn wound is also characteristic of invasive pseudomonas burn wound infection, but edema and erythematous discoloration of the unburned skin at the wound margin, producing an exaggerated "step-

---

* The opinions or assertions contained herein are the private views of the authors and are not to be construed as official or as reflecting the views of the Department of the Army or the Department of Defense.

Table 1. Clinical signs of invasive burn wound infection

I.	Dark brown, or violaceous discoloration of the burn wound: can be focal, multifocal or generalized.
II.	Conversion of partial-thickness injury to full-thickness necrosis.
III.	Hemorrhagic discoloration of subeschar tissue.
IV.	Green pigment visible in subcutaneous fat.
V.	Erythematous nodular lesions (ecthyma gangrenosum) in unburned skin.
VI.	Edema and/or violaceous discoloration of unburned skin at wound margins.
VII.	Unexpectedly rapid separation of eschar: most commonly due to fungal infection.
VIII.	Rapid centrifugal advance of subcutaneous edema with central ischemic necrosis: typical of *Phycomycotic* infection.
IX.	Vesicular lesions in healing or healed second-degree burns*
X.	Crusted serrated margins of partial-thickness burns of face*

* Characteristic of herpetic infection

off" between intact skin surface and burn wound bed are generic changes indicative of nonspecific infection.

Other organism-specific changes include the dusky discoloration of saponified subcutaneous fat often associated with invasive fungal infection, and the vesicular lesions in healing or healed partial-thickness burns and the crusted serrated margins of partial-thickness burns, particularly those in the nasolabial area of the face that are virtually pathognomonic of herpes simplex virus infections [1].

The unreliability and lack of specificity of local signs and symptoms require that other methods be used to assess the microbial status of the burn wound and diagnose burn wound infections. Surface culture techniques may be used for epidemiologic monitoring and to determine the predominant flora of the burn wounds of individual patients, but the frequent surface microbial colonization of burn wounds and the failure of such cultures to sample the subeschar space make them ineffectual in diagnosing burn wound infection. Cultures of burn wound tissue can provide a more precise assessment of burn wound microbial ecology and dynamics.

During the period 1 January 1987 through 27 December 1991, cultures were performed on 2158 burn wound tissue samples (biopsies plus surgical specimens) removed from 501 of the 1080 burn patients admitted during that period. Six-hundred and sixty-five, or 31%, of the biopsies that were removed from 210, or 42%, of those patients showed microbial growth. Isolates recovered from 144 patients were positive for bacteria while isolates recovered from 44 patients were positive for yeasts, and isolates recovered from 130 patients were positive for filamentous fungi. Recovery of bacteria, in order of decreasing frequency, consisted of: *Staphylococcus aureus* from 45 patients, *Pseudomonas aeruginosa* from 36 patients, *E. coli* from 28 patients, *Enterococci* from 20 patients, *Klebsiella pneumoniae* from 11 patients, *Bacillus* species from 18 patients, and *Enterobacter cloacae* from 14 patients. Recovery of yeasts consisted of: *Candida albicans* from 29 patients, *Candida rugosa* from seven patients, and *Candida tropicalis* from three patients. The recovery of filamentous fungi consisted of *Aspergillus* species from 59 patients, *Fusarium* species from 11 patients, *Cladosporium* species from nine patients, *Penicillium* species from seven patients, and *Phycomycetes* (mucor species and rhizopus species) from three pa-

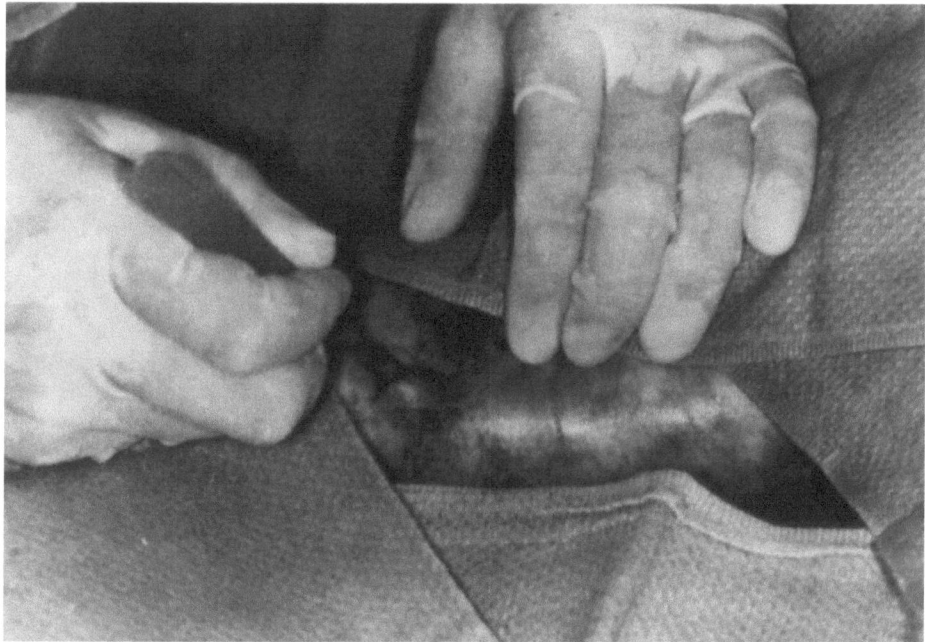

Fig. 1. The scalpel is used to biopsy the burn wound at a site selected on the basis of dark hemorrhagic discoloration as shown here. Note the depth to which the scalpel blade has been inserted to insure that unburned subcutaneous tissue will be included in the biopsy

tients. Such surveillance-type culture data are of assistance in monitoring the ecological changes that occur in the indigenous burn wound flora of a burn unit across time and in selecting agents for initial systemic antimicrobial therapy in patients who do develop an invasive infection. Systemic therapy is subsequently altered as necessary based upon culture and sensitivity of the organisms causing a specific infection. Such epidemiologic information is also useful in identifying the need to modify infection control measures to eliminate environmental or other vectors responsible for cross contamination and prevent the establishment of resistant endemic strains in a treatment facility.

Burn wound biopsies can be used to obtain quantitative culture data and perform a histologic examination of both the eschar and the subeschar tissue. To prepare the wound for a biopsy, that area of the burn showing the most pronounced tinctorial and morphologic changes should be cleansed to remove debris and residual topical agent. Following cleansing, a lenticular 500-mg tissue sample that includes eschar and underlying unburned subcutaneous tissue is obtained by use of the scapel (Fig. 1). If local anesthesia is necessary, the anesthetic agent should be injected at the periphery of the planned sampling site to avoid distortion of the architecture of the specimen. The specimen is bisected and one-half is processed in the microbiology laboratory to identify the organisms present and to characterize the predominant members of the microbial flora. Although recommended by some, quantitative cultures are unreliable in diagnosing burn wound infection [8]. Falsely high quantitative counts can result from culturing pooled secretions or exudates, culturing an eschar at the time of slough that occurs as a result of bacterial proliferation at the nonviable tissue interface, or from delay in specimen transport that permits in vitro microbial proliferation. Conversely, falsely low quantitative culture counts can result from culturing a non-representative desiccated area of the wound, culturing residual topical agent, and storage or transport conditions that allow the specimen to desiccate.

Studies by McManus et al. have shown that quantitative cultures are clinically useful only to confirm the absence of invasive infection, i.e., low microbial counts are seldom associated with histologic evidence of invasive infection. The natural history of a full-thickness burn wound entails a progressive increase in microbial density, particularly at the subeschar interface between viable and nonviable tissue (where the organisms contribute to collagenolysis and sloughing of the nonviable tissue) with proliferation enhanced by maceration and pooling of wound exudate. Consequently, quantitative counts of more than 10^5 organisms per gram of tissue in a biopsy specimen (the density claimed by some to be diagnostic of invasive infection) are actually unreliable and correlate with histologic evidence of invasive burn wound infection in less than 50% of biopsies [5]. In short, the histologic examination of a biopsy specimen harvested from an area of the burn wound suspected of harboring infection has a shorter turnaround time than culture techniques; it is the only accurate means of differentiating colonization of nonviable eschar (always present to some degree) from invasion of viable tissue and making a reliable diagnosis of invasive burn wound infection, and can readily identify infections caused by fungi and viruses for which cultures are of little clinical usefulness.

Accordingly, the other half of the biopsy specimen is processed by either a rapid section technique that requires 3 to 4 hours for slide preparation or by a frozen-section technique that requires only 30 min for slide preparation [3, 4]. Since the frozen-section technique is associated with a falsely negative rate of 3.6%, the biopsy sample should be processed by standard techniques to confirm frozen section diagnosis and exclude falsely negative frozen section readings. The pathologist examines the sections looking for the histologic signs of burn wound infection listed in Table 2. The identification of bacteria, fungi, or viruses in viable tissue in the histologic section confirms the diagnosis of invasive burn wound infection. The other histologic criteria indicative of burn wound infection may be found in association with inflammation, but their presence should heighten one's index of suspicion and prompt a careful search for microorganisms. Both falsely negative and falsely positive biopsy readings may occur. A falsely positive reading may be caused by artifacts produced

Table 2. Histopathologic signs of burn wound infection

I.	Microorganisms present in unburned tissue.
II.	Heightened inflammatory reaction in unburned tissue.
III.	Hemorrhage in unburned tissue.
IV.	Small vessel thrombosis and ischemic necrosis of unburned tissue.
V.	Dense microbial growth in subeschar space and along hair follicles and sweat glands.
VI.	Intracellular viral inclusions A. Type-A Cowdry bodies B. Intracellular virions

Table 3. Histologic staging of burn wound microbial status

Stage		Characteristics
I.	Colonization	
	A. Superficial	Microorganisms present on burn wound surface
	B. Penetration	Microorganisms present in variable thickness of the eschar
	C. Proliferation	Variable density of microorganisms in subeschar space
II.	Invasion	
	A. Microinvasion	Microscopic foci of microorganisms in viable tissue adjacent to subeschar space
	B. Generalized	Multifocal or wide-spread penetration of microorganisms deep into viable subcutaneous tissue
	C. Microvascular	Involvement of small blood vessels and lymphatics

by tissue processing or adherence of foreign bodies or as the result of misinterpretation by an inexperienced pathologist. Falsely negative readings can occur as a result of inadequate tissue dehydration, excessive thickness of the histologic sections, inadequate sampling (biopsy of an uninfected site or sampling of only the eschar without attached unburned tissue), and misinterpretation of histologic findings by an inexperienced pathologist.

A grading scheme has been developed to classify the microbial status of biopsy specimens on the basis of histologic evidence of microbial density and penetration (Table 3) [13]. As is immediately evident, the important differentiation is between Stage IC, colonization with penetration of the full-thickness of the eschar und proliferation at the viable/nonviable tissue interface, and Stage IIA, microinvasion of viable tissue which confirms the presence of an invasive burn wound infection (Fig. 2). Mortality increases as histologic staging designation increases, i.e., the risk of remote spread and mortality associated with a Stage II classification is greater than that associated with Stage I disease. The occurrence of mortality in patients with Stage I biopsy findings appears to be related to other complications in patients from whom the eschar cannot be excised and the wound closed prior to full-thickness penetration of the microorganisms. The striking difference in the mortality associated with Stages IC and IIA reflects the impact of invasive infection on burn patient outcome. A histologic staging of IIC with microvascular and lymphathic involvement is associated with a high incidence of microbial recovery from the blood, dissemination of the infection to remote tissues and organs, and an almost universal mortality (Fig. 3) [11].

The histologic findings in a burn wound biopsy must always be interpreted in light of the patient's clinical status and trajectory. A negative reading of a biopsy obtained from a patient with progressive expansion in the size or number of wound areas showing tinctorial or morphologic change consistent with infection demands additional biopsies of those areas. Those occasional patients who show clinical deterioration consistent with sepsis and whose wounds show rapid, dark discoloration consistent with accelerated maturation should have serial biopsies performed and, if progressive increase in the stage of the successive biopsies is noted, wound care should be altered to use only sulfamylon topical chemotherapy and effect surgical excision of the involved tissue as soon as the patient's general condition permits.

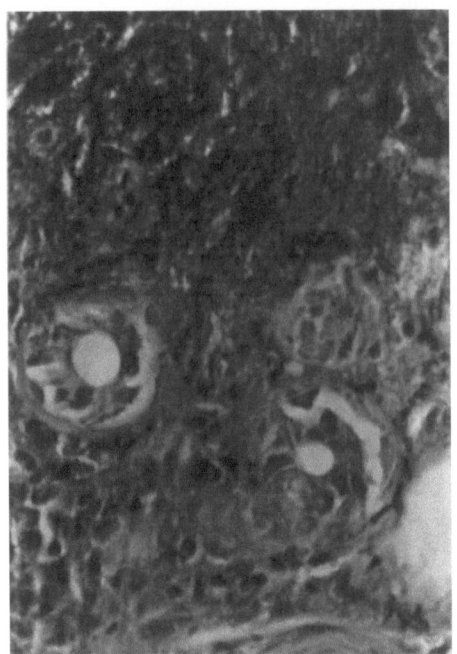

Fig. 2. This histologic section from a burn wound biopsy shows dark staining masses of bacillary organisms in the upper half of the section extending into unburned tissue: Stage IIA invasive infection

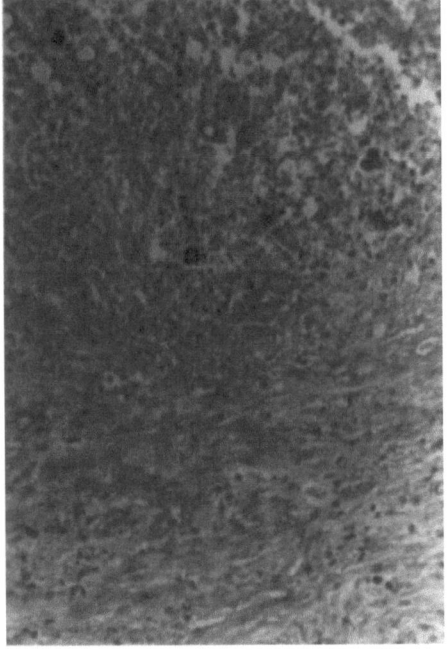

Fig. 3. This histologic section from a burn wound biopsy shows fungal elements and marked inflammatory changes within the lumen of an involved microvessel: Stage IIC invasive infection

During the period January 1987 through December 1991, the burn wounds of 178 patients treated at this Institute underwent biopsy. The biopsies from 67 patients were reported by the pathologist as being histologically negative, i.e., organisms may not be visible when the microbial density is less than 10^5 per gram of tissue. The biopsies from 85 patients showed only colonization, i.e., Stages IA–IC, and the biopsies from 26 patients were reported as showing invasive burn wound infection, i.e., Stages IIA–IIC. In 18 patients the infecting organisms were filamentous fungi, *Aspergillus* species in 16 and *Mucor* species in two, and in four patients *Candida* species were the causative organisms. In four patients bacteria were the infecting organisms, *Pseudomonas aeruginosa* in two, *Staphylococcus aureus* in one and group D *Enterococcus* in one. The current predominance of nonbacterial burn wound infections and the relative rarity of gram-negative bacillary burn wound infections emphasize the utility of histologic examination by which one can readily identify invading fungi. The mean age of the 26 patients in whom invasive burn wound infection was diagnosed in a biopsy specimen obtained on the basis of clinical suspicion was 41.3 years, and the mean total extent of burn was 56.6% of the total body surface with 45.1% being full-thickness burn. The invasive wound infection was diagnosed as early as the seventh postburn day and as late as the 56th postburn day, with the mean time of diagnosis being the 22nd postburn day. Eighteen, or 60%, of those patients died.

The mean age of the 18 patients with wound infections caused by filamentous fungi was 38.2 years and the mean total extent of burn was 66% of the total body surface. Twelve, or 75%, of the 16 patients with *Aspergillus* wound infections died but, somewhat surprisingly, both of the patients with mucor species infection survived. The average extent of burn (67.3%) in the patients who died with invasive fungal infection was not statistically different from the size of burn (64%) in the patients who survived, but the effect of age on both burn and infection related mortality was evident; the average age of those patients with filamentous fungal infections who died was 44 years, vs. an average of 27 years for those patients who survived both the fungal infection and their burn. In four patients in whom an initial burn wound biopsy showed some gradation of Stage-I colonization, a repeat biopsy 2 to 11 days later at another site revealed invasive *Aspergillus* infection. The diagnosis of wound invasion prompted immediate excision of the infected tissue. The survival of two (50%) of those patients emphasizes the importance of early diagnosis made possible by biopsy monitoring.

There were four patients in whom *Candida* was the cause of invasive burn wound infection and three (75%) of those patients expired. The average extent of burn in those patients was only 27% of the total body surface, but the average age was 72 years. The average time of death of the three patients with *Candida* infection who expired was the 58th postburn day. There were four additional patients in whom bacteria were the cause of invasive burn wound infection and three, or 75%, of those patients expired. The mean age of the patients who developed bacterial burn wound infection was 24 years, the average extent of burn was 43% of the total body surface, and the average time of death was the 22nd postburn day.

Twenty of the entire group of 26 patients with histologically confirmed invasive burn wound infection underwent excision of the infected wound as soon as they could be prepared for surgery: an average of 2.4 days after biopsy. The other six patients who had burn wound infections were so physiologically unstable that excision could not be performed and they expired on an average of 6 days after biopsy

Table 4. Biopsy microbial status and patient outcome

Biopsy stage	Survivors	Deaths	Mortality rate
IIA	7	13	65%
IIB and IIC	1	5	83%

(range day of biopsy to 15 days postbiopsy). In all of those six patients invasive burn wound infection was present and was considered to be a contributing factor to the patient's demise. In only two patients was the infection considered to be the principal cause of death. Even in this small group of patients, histologic stage of invasion was related to outcome. Six (35%) of the 20 patients with Stage IIA infections survived while only one (17%) of the patients with Stages IIB or IIC infections survived (Table 4).

There were an additional 16 patients in whom invasive infection was diagnosed as an incidental finding in surgical specimens. Six of these 16 patients expired. In five patients, burn wound infection was present at the time of death and was considered to be a contributing factor in the patient's demise. In the other patient, autopsy examination revealed no burn wound infection. The fact that only six, or 38%, of those 16 patients expired emphasizes the importance of early excision of infected burns before the infection produces wound changes or systemic signs.

Tissue biopsies can also be used to confirm depth of a burn wound, i.e., differentiate partial-thickness from full-thickness burns; assess adequacy of debridement of electric injury or an infected burn wound, i.e., differentiate viable from nonviable tissue; diagnose suppurative thrombophlebitis, i.e., differentiate thrombosis from intraluminal infection [14]; diagnose disseminated intravascular coagulation (DIC), i.e., differentiate hemorrhagic change due to local trauma from petechia due to coagulopathy; and diagnose exfoliative skin diseases, i.e., differentiate idiosyncratic or hypersensitivity related exfoliative dermatitides from *Staphylococcal* scalded skin syndrome [2]. During the time period covered by this review, tissue biopsies were used for all those purposes except for diagnosis of burn depth, a use obviated by early burn wound excision, and for diagnosis of DIC, a use obviated by availability of accurate laboratory tests.

There were 11 patients from whom segments of 13 previously cannulated veins were biopsied because of a suspicion of suppurative thrombophlebitis in the absence of gross intraluminal suppuration. In two patients fungal suppurative thrombophlebitis was histologically documented with *Aspergillus* identified in one saphenous vein and *Aspergillus* plus *Candida* in a forearm vein. Identification of the intraluminal infection prompted immediate excision of the infected vein in both patients. The excision controlled the septic process and both patients survived.

During the same time period, 85 wound biopsies were performed in 27 patients to characterize and diagnose exfoliative dermatitic processes. In 24 patients, toxic epidermal necrolysis (TEN) was confirmed and differentiated from *Staphylococcal* scalded skin syndrome, which was present in only two patients. There was one patient in whom the dermatitic change was due to an allergic reaction. In one of the ten patients, Stage IIA *Aspergillus* species wound invasion of the face was identified as a preterminal complication. Both of the patients with *Staphylococcal* scalded skin syndrome survived, and 18 of the 24 TEN patients survived.

The use of burn wound biopsies to assess the microbial status of the burn wound and differentiate invasive burn wound infection from microbial colonization of an eschar permits timely intervention to control the infection and increase the patient's likelihood of survival. The use of wound biopsies to differentiate burn depth, assess the adequacy of tissue debridement, and diagnose a variety of infectious and inflammatory conditions enables the attending surgeon to tailor therapeutic interventions, both surgical and pharmacologic, to meet the individual patient's needs and treat documented complications appropriately.

References

1. Foley FD, Greenwald KA, Nash G, Pruitt BA Jr (1970) Herpesvirus infection in burn patients. N Engl J Med 282:652–656
2. Halebian PH, Madden MR, Finklestein JL (1986) Improved burn center survival of patients with toxic epidermal necrolysis managed without corticosteroids. Ann Surg 204:503–512
3. Kim SH, Hubbard GB, McManus WF (1985) Frozen section technique to evaluate early burn wound biopsy: A comparison with the rapid section technique. J Trauma 25:1134–1137
4. Kim SH, Hubbard GB, Worley BL (1985) A rapid section technique for burn wound biopsy. J Burn Care Rehab 6:433–435
5. McManus AT, Kim SH, McManus WF (1987) Comparison of quantitative microbiology and histopathology in divided burn wound biopsy specimens. Arch Surg 122:74–76
6. Pruitt BA Jr (1984) The diagnosis and treatment of infection in the burn patient. Burns 11:79–91
7. Pruitt BA Jr (1984) Phycomycotic infections. Problems in General Surgery (ed Alexander JW). J.B. Lippincott Company, Philadelphia, pp 664–678
8. Pruitt BA Jr (1986) Host-opportunist interactions in surgical infections. Arch Surg 121:13–22
9. Pruitt BA Jr (1987) Infection: Cause or effect of pathophysiologic change in burn and trauma patients. In: Lipid Mediators in the Immunology of Shock (M. Paubert-Braquet) (Ed.). Plenum Press, New York, pp 31–42
10. Pruitt BA Jr, Curreri PW (1971) The burn wound and its care. Arch Surg 130:461–468
11. Pruitt BA Jr, Foley FD (1973) The use of biopsies in burn patient care. Surgery 73:887–897
12. Pruitt BA Jr, Goodwin CW (1987) Thermal injuries. In Clinical Surgery (ed Davis JH). C.V. Mosby Company, St Louis, pp 2861
13. Pruitt BA Jr and Goodwin CW (1987) Thermal injuries. In Clinical Surgery (ed Davis JH). C.V. Mosby Company, St Louis, pp 2863–2866
14. Pruitt BA Jr, McManus WF, Kim SH (1980) Diagnosis and treatment of cannula related intravenous sepsis in burn patients. Ann Surg 191:546–544

Authors' address:
B.A. Pruitt Jr., M.D., F.A.C.S.
Colonel, MC
US Army Institute of Surgical Research
Fort Sam Houston, Texas 78234-5012
USA

The problem of lung infection in extensive burns

J. Guilbaud and Y. Legulluche

Hôpital d'Instruction des Armées Percy, Clamart, France

Prior to the use of effective topical antimicrobial therapy, infection of the burn wound was the leading cause of mortality in patients with extensive burns. Actually, pneumonia is the most frequent life-threatening infection encountered in burn patients. The burn patient is an ideal, fully designated victim to present infectious pulmonary complications:

Depressed systemic host defenses, infection of the burn wound with resultant toxemia and bacteremia, pulmonary alterations due to burns both with inhalation injury or primary lesions of the respiratory tract (burns, soot, blast injury) which can directly impair lung defenses, oropharyngeal colonization are many factors which may contribute to the development of infectious pulmonary complications in the burned patient.

The burn patient is an immunodepressed patient

Extensive burn injuries – greater than 40% TBSA – profoundly depress the host defense mechanisms and predispose the patients to systemic infections. The effects of burn injury on host defenses are:

A depression of cell-mediated immunity:

The principal T-cell abnormalities are T-cell lymphopenia with a significant reduction in the T4/T8 ratio. The depression in the T-cell function is marked by reduced in vitro-cytotoxicity, decreased lymphoprofilerative responses, extensive T-suppressor cell activity, defective natural killer activity and decreased lymphokine production with a significantly depressed ability to produce IL2. The absolute number of suppressor T-cells is increased in patients with burns >25% TBSA. When incubated in the presence of serum from thermally injured patients, normal T-lymphocytes can become non specific T-lymphocytes.

A suppression of phagocyte functions

There are numerous reports demonstrating that polymorphonuclear leukocytes (PMN) from severely burned patients exhibit reduced chemotactic responses, compromised phagocytosis, and decreased intracellular bactericidal capacity. Thus, the ability of circulating leucocytic phagocytes to emigrate to extravascular sites of infection – such as the lung is impaired. Various functions of PMN including aggregation, chemotaxis, superoxyde production, and lysosomal enzyme release have been shown to be inhibited by PGE1 and PGE2, primary products of arachidonic acid metabolism via the cyclooxygenase pathway.

The defects in phagocyte function following burn injury are probably a consequence of their exposure to abnormal stimuli, rending the phagocyte refractory to further stimulation, thus creating an impaired capacity to respond to a second, localized infected site such as the lung.

The release of immunosuppressive mediators

Immunosuppressive substances are present in the sera of patients with burns and are directly related to the extent of burn injury: arachidonic acid metabolites, cytokines, endotoxins, glucocorticoids.

A depletion of the complement system

Burn injury results in an immediate and dramatic fall in alternate complement pathway due to a massive activation, as shown by the presence of complement cleavage products and the occurrence of immune complexes. The complement cleavage products can produce a series of changes of cell-mediated immune functions. C3a binds preferentially to eosinophils and basophils and induces histamine release from basophils and mast cells. It inhibits specific antibody responses. C3a and C5a increase vascular permeability. C5a promotes the aggregation and adhesiveness of circulating neutrophils, resulting in the formation of microemboli which are sequestered in the small vessels of the pulmonary circulation and can induce both pulmonary hypertension and arterial hypoxemia.

A depletion of immunoglobulin

Depletion of immunoglobulin by increased consumption and depletion of serum opsonic activity: opsonins are factors which stimulate phagocytosis and render bacteria more susceptible to phagocytic uptake by neutrophils and macrophages. A transient depression in B-lymphocyte cell population and immunoglobulin production follows burns injuries. An increase in the clearance and/or catabolism of serum antibody together with a normal or even elevated synthesis could be one mechanism for depressed serum levels. These defects in host defense mechanisms provide a potential mechanism for the clinical association of burn injury, sepsis, and pneumonia [36].

The burn wound is a constant source of bacteria release

The burn eschar is a constant starting point for bacteria release in spite of effective topical chemotherapy. Both wound factors and microbial factors influence the rate of proliferation and the balance between host defense capability; the capacity of the bacterial population of the wound to spread determines whether infection will occur.

The denatured proteins of the burn eschar serve as an excellent culture medium to support the growth and proliferation of the colonizing micro-organisms. Moreover, the avascularity of the burned tissue limits the delivery of both endogenous and exogenous antibacterial agents to the site of microbial proliferation. Thus, the burn wound can be a reservoir for bacteria release.

Even without direct pulmonary damage, the lung of the burn patient is not normal

Burn injury not only causes skin damage and tissue necrosis but also exerts deleterious effects on every organ system. There are lung alterations associated with pure thermal damage to the dermis: they include an increase in lung lymph flow and edema formation, a transient pulmonary hypertension and a decrease in PaO_2 together with a significant decrease in lung compliance. Different mechanisms have been proposed to explain these alterations. Numerous authors have reported that a number of vaso-active mediators, including thromboxane A2, histamine, serotonin together with bacterial byproducts are released from the burn tissue and both compromise the pulmonary vasculature and have an effect on smooth muscle constriction in the lung [11]. TxA2 produces vaso-constriction, raising pulmonary pressure and increases broncho-constriction, causing decreased lung compliance due to increased air-way resistance. Serotonin produces pulmonary vaso-constriction. Thus, the good ratio between lung perfusion and lung ventilation for providing adequate gas exchange is impaired. The treatment itself can add its own effects: in the absence of protein for resuscitation there is an increase in lung transvascular fluid flux as measured by lymph flow, probably due to the degree of hypoproteinemia. Additionally, pulmonary capillary blood flow is increased after resuscitation because of the increase in cardiac output. This increase in pulmonary capillary perfusion could increase edema formation. On the other hand, products of sequestered neutrophils such as oxygen free radicals and proteases destroy the endothelial layer as well as the interstitium; they could cause a possible increase in fluid and protein leakage into the interstitium and alveoli. As to whether pulmonary edema is seen following burn injuries is controversial [16]. Certain authors such as Demling, have denied the existence of edema formation as there is no increase in measured lung water. These lesions with pure thermal injury are seldom manifested clinically, but these microvascular changes make the lung more sensitive to septic insults and smoke inhalation.

Furthermore, the wound creates an increase in tissue oxygen requirement. As a result of hypermetabolism, the increased carbon-dioxide component induces a strong demand on the lung for increased minute ventilation with subsequent decrease in tidal volume which can greatly potentiate any underlying pulmonary injury. The decrease in tidal volume can also be due to a constrictive eschar. Hyperventilation due to pain may also lead to the same situation. All these changes in lung compliance, oxygen delivery and oxygen demand can occur without inhalation injury.

Lung can be directly damaged by primary respiratory lesions

The presence or the absence of primary lesions of the lungs may be a stronger determinant of mortality than the size of the burn injury. The incidence of inhalation injury (II) varies according to the authors between 15 and 33 % (Nelson) of all thermally injured patients admitted to the burn units. Bronchopneumonia appears in 15 to 60 % of these patients (and has a reported mortality rate of 50 to 80 %). Reviewing the records of more than 1000 patients treated at a single institution, Pruitt has found that 38 % of the patients with II had subsequent pneumonia while only 8.8 % of the patients without II had a pneumonia [35].

In healthy individuals, the invading pathogens encounter a system of defense mechanism composed of both mechanical defenses for the upper airway and cellular and chemical defenses for the alveoli. There are five major defense mechanisms:

- aerodynamic filtration;
- mucociliary system;
- airway reflexes (cough, bronchospasm);
- soluble factors in airway secretions;
- phagocytic cells.

The majority of pulmonary problems that result from II are caused by chemical irritants such as aldehydes, while burn lesions due to inhalation of heated air are confined to the face, and to the oropharynx and upper airway, which thermoregulate, humidify, and filter inhaled air.

The tracheobronchial area can be damaged by irritants which can produce changes similar to those seen after exposure to acids. The volatile gases can cause a halt in cilia functioning, resulting in impaired mucus clearance [40].

Free radicals have been reported to be present in smoke and have been implicated in edema formation by way of changes in microvascular permeability and increased microvascular pressure. A substantial increase in blood flow to the tracheobronchial area probably due to the release of vasoactive polypeptides (TxA2) and/or histamine contributes to the formation of exudate and edema. The protein-rich plasma exudation into the trachebronchial tree may serve as a medium for bacterial growth. Bronchospasm frequently occurs and the resultant airway obstruction combined with retained secretions further impairs the effective pulmonary cleaning process, increasing susceptibility to lung infections. Moreover, the damaged epithelium forms pseudomembranous casts, causing an obstruction of the airway with areas of atelectasis.

At the lung level, insufflation of only one lung with smoke is followed by a marked shunting of blood flow and, therefore, by changes in the ventilation/perfusion ratio which leads to an early fall in arterial oxygenation and in the formation of which the products of cyclooxygenase pathway have their responsibility [21]. Wu et al. have reported normalization of acute changes in this ratio following inhalation injury by treatment with cyclooxygenase inhibitors.

In spite of controversial findings between studies by Clark and Prien, it is reasonable to think that damage to the epithelial areas in the alveoli includes the alveolar type II cells which are responsible for the synthesis of surfactant materials. This may also contribute to the development of peripheral atelectasis. Chemical irritants induce an activation of alveolar macrophages (AM) which mediates an influx of PMN into the lung. These neutrophils produce high concentrations of proteolytic enzymes such as trypsin and elastase into the lung which can contribute, together with oxygen-free radicals, to the severity of pulmonary complications [18, 19]. At the same time, the antibacterial properties of AM should be adversely affected with a diminished phagocytic potential, a decrease in adherence and a decrease in their bactericidal functions.

In the Pruitt's investigation, II alone increased mortality by 20 % and pneumonia by 40 %, with a maximum increase of approximately 60 % when both were present. Thus, all conditions are gathered to allow septic complications and particularly to allow pneumonia to occur.

Burn patient presents a maximum risk factor for nosocomial pneumonia

Procedures commonly employed in the management of critically ill patients can have adverse effects on the patient's antibacterial defenses. Nasogastric tubes for continuous enteral feeding and early intubation for airway management and ventilatory support are frequently utilized in burn patients [9]. Patients receiving mechanical ventilation have a fourfold increase in risk for hospital acquired pneumonia. The origin of the bacteria infecting the lungs is twofold: mainly endogenous (digestive tract) and exogenous. The most common mechanism in the development of pneumonia is the endogenous colonization of the oropharynx followed by aspiration of bacteria into the lungs of a patient whose normal antibacterial defenses have been impaired. Naso-oropharyngeal flora carries 2 to 10% of gram-negative bacteria (GNB). In hospitalized patients it enriches rapidly up to 75% with GNB and the oropharynx becomes a reservoir for gramnegative bacteria [7].

The routine neutralization of gastric acidity by H_2 blockers and antacids raises gastric pH and allows overgrowth of gram-negative in the stomach, and retrograde movement of bacteria from the stomach to the oropharynx can occur, the presence of nasogastric tubes facilitating their migration [3]. The nasogastric tube may also alter the esophagal sphincters and esophagal motricity with reflux coming from the gastro-intestinal tract. From the pharynx the nose is rapidly colonized and the presence of foreign material in the nostrils favors infection of the facial pneumatic cavities (maxillary, ethmoidal and sphenoidal sinus). After a few days of intubation, more than ⅔ of the patients have contracted bacterial sinusitis. Endotracheal tubes disrupt and bypass the normal epiglottic function, impair the ciliary escalator and the cough mechanism, and allow bacteria to migrate around the cuff from oropharynx into the lungs [8]. Dumoulin was the first to document a change in gastric bacteriology by quantitative techniques and to show a direct correlation between gastric pH and the bacterial flora from zero at a pH of 1 to $>10^7$ cfu/ml at a pH of 6.0 in patients receiving antacids or cimetidine. In the prospective study of Freiburg the occurrence of pneumonia correlates directly with an increase in the gastric pH: the disease occurred at a rate of 40 % when the pH was < 3.4 vs 70 % when the pH was > 5.

Several other factors contribute to alter the oropharyngeal flora:

– Antibiotherapy selects for or promotes the growth of more resistant bacteria which may then either become colonizing or infecting pathogens. Furthermore, antibiotics are known to increase the ability of gram-negative to adhere to the oropharynx.
– Steroid treatment is associated with more infectious complications such as pneumonia and bacteremia. In a study by Moylan of patients with documented inhalation injury, the steroid treatment was associated with an increased mortality rate (53 % vs 12 %).

– Narcotics, hypnotics, and neuroleptics predispose the patient to aspiration by altering his/her level of consciousness and by depressing the cough reflex [15].

Available data show a predominant rate for gram-negative bacteria and staphylococci in pneumonia [2]. (*P. aeruginosa* is the single most frequently isolated pathogen, with various members of the family *Enterobacteriaceae. Acinetobacter calcoaceticus var. Anitratus* also emerge as a significant pathogen in some centers.)

Exogenous sources are essentially respiratory equipment [26] or the hands of the staff. In a prospective study, Cross and Roy have shown that in only a small portion of patients on respiratory devices can contaminated devices be directly implicated as the source of infection. In some instances, bacteria may invade the lung by way of hematogenous spread from a site of infection elsewhere. However, in a recent study Mock reports that in nine of the 10 patients who actually had pneumonia, positive sputum cultures preceded positive blood cultures for the same organism. This argues strongly that, "in patients who have pneumonia", the organisms first enter the tracheobronchial tree and infiltrate the parenchyma of the lung, then enter the blood stream (Kenneth Burchard).

Diagnosis

Prompt diagnosis is particularly important because the mortality rate associated with lung infection in these immunodepressed patients may be as high as 40%.

The combination of clinical and laboratory parameters, positive bacterial findings and appropriate appearance of roentgenography of the chest are the best indication of the presence of lung infection.

Clinical diagnosis

New and persistent radiographic infiltrates, fever and shivers or hypothermia, leukocytosis or leukopenia, purulent tracheobronchial secretions and impairment of gas exchanges or impairment of respiratory requirements are the diagnostic criteria most frequently used in mechanically ventilated patients. However, they are non-specific and, in the case of A.R.D.S., have a low sensitivity [22]. Furthermore, fever and leukocytosis as a result of other disease processes may specially appear in the burn patient, and the analysis of tracheobronchial secretions frequently indicates the presence of pneumonia when no pneumonia is present. None of these signs taken independently has any sufficient positive predictable value and their absence does not eliminate a pneumopathy under mechanical ventilation. Some respiratory signs such as dyspnea, cyanosis, thoracic pain, hemoptysia, and cough appear more often in non-ventilated patients. Neuro-psychic and digestive troubles cannot easily be attributed to pulmonary damage.

Even when clinical, radiological, and biological data are present, they require bacteriological confirmation of acquired pneumopathy.

Radiological diagnosis

Both physical findings and the chest radiograph are difficult to interpret in a population where obstructive pulmonary disease, congestive heart failure, and A.R.D.S. may also be present [31]. Pulmonary infiltrates may be hidden by an edema, or may represent atelectasis, pulmonary edema or pulmonary contusions in patients who have experienced trauma. That is the reason why the radiological diagnosis is difficult and why clinicians may either underdiagnose or overdiagnose pneumonia. In cases where there is not a serious emergency, when the lung was previously healthy, the key to the diagnosis is radiological: apparition and persistence for at least 24 h of a new parenchymal infiltrate or change in a preexisting anomaly considered as being minor. This time allows to start techniques devoted to fight against ventilatory disorders or to eliminate pleural pathology, localized edema or pulmonary infarction. Nevertheless, distinguishing nosocomial pneumonia (NP) from purulent tracheobronchitis may be difficult.

One study that compared the clinical diagnosis of NP with histopathologic evidence of autopsy in patients with A.R.D.S. found that pneumonia was misdiagnosed 30% of the time. In a similar report Bell found evidence of pneumonia in 26% of the cases.

Among diagnostic imaging techniques, chest radiography remains the single most common imaging examination [38]. A standard chest X-ray will be performed every 24 h in the same position (dorsal decubitus or seated) and with comparable parameters.

Computed tomography (CT) (tomodensitometry) performed with 60 to 120 ml of contrast product is always achievable in an intubated and mechanically ventilated patient. Standard chest x-rays are sometimes defective and occasionally only the CT will bring out the pulmonary disorder [14].

Therefore, a good indication for performing the CT examination is the existence of a clinical chart which leads to a diagnosis of pneumopathy such as fever, leucocytosis, purulent aspiration, without a precise radiological image (A.R.D.S., pulmonary contusion, chronic bronchopathy).

- Magnetic resonance imaging is extremely difficult because most support apparatus (mechanical ventilators, infusion pumps, etc.) are ferromagnetic.
- Echography helps to determine the liquid and/or the parenchymal part of a visible opacity on the pulmonary x-ray.
- Computed angiography could allow to eliminate an embolical migration, whose diagnosis is sometimes difficult to exclude in the presence of a focal pneumopathy [20, 30].

Mock, Burchard, et al. have proposed a scoring system that incorporates roentgenographic information and which should give the best predictive diagnosis. The scoring system assigns one point each for: presence of new infiltrate, acinar shadows, air bronchograms, segmental or asymmetric infiltrates, infiltrates in non-dependent portions of lung and ipsilateral pleural effusion in association with a new infiltrate on a roentgenogram of the chest, absence of volume loss, absence of cardiomegaly and absence of hilar enlargement. A total score of 0 to 3 indicates non-pneumonia, 4 to 7 indicates moderate probability, and higher than 7 indicates a high probability of pneumonia.

Bacteriological diagnosis

Etiologic diagnosis is difficult as a result of the difficulty to differentitate colonizing and infecting pathogens, all the more so since there is a straight correlation between this colonization and lung parenchymal infection.

The occurrence of pneumonia due to a single organism while multiple pathogens colonize the proximal airways is explained by the process of selection by lung defenses. Infections are caused by organisms most able to evade defenses. Polymicrobial pneumonia generally implies a more serious deficiency in host defenses. The appearance of a pulmonary infiltrate together with obtaining positive hemocultures have a strong orientation value; obtaining bacterias by pleural puncture or by the puncture of an abcess give a definite diagnosis. The theoretical reference is lung biopsy with culture [4]. Nevertheless, ordinarily, bacteriological diagnosis imposes to resort to an endobronchial investigation. Sample techniques are either qualitative and aim at identifying the bacteria or the bacterias responsible for infection, or quantitative, thus allowing, not only to identify responsible germs, but also to overturn a diagnosis of presumption into a diagnosis of certainty.

It is therefore necessary to make a distinction between colonization and infection. This is possible thanks to the methods aimed at obtaining a distal and protected sample; in most cases, the sample will be directed.

Except in rather rare cases where a bacterial sample is possible from the puncture of an homolateral pleuresia or of a pulmonary abscess, the diagnosis of pneumonia with certainty relies on bacteriological and, eventually, histological characteristics of the infected lung. Sampling and examination of the liquid of tracheal suction is the easiest method [3]. Not very specific, it allows, in the absence of germs in the direct examination and in the culture, to invalidate the diagnosis of pneumonia [4, 25].

Two techniques, bronchoalveolar lavage (BAL) and protected specimen brushing (PSB) have been used to obtain samples in distal lung [5].

- BAL performed with a cuffed catheter or with a fiber-optic bronchoscope samples a large surface of the lung and allows a rapid diagnostic and a therapeutic orientation. The % of intracellular bacteria is estimated from 300 cells and one can assert the presence of an acquired pneumonia if $\geq 5\%$ of the cells contain intracellular bacteria [6].
  The possible diffusion of the infectious process could be an inconvenience. In patients with diffuse infiltrates and a worsening clinical course, BAL provides the better sampling of the lung's flora. BAL is less specific, but more sensitive than PSB.
- PSB is an excellent diagnostic examination. It has the greatest specificity for predicting future course ($>95\%$). A value of $>10^3$ cfu/ml appears to be a reliable indicator of clinically important pneumonia [13]. PSB collecting about 0.01 ml of fluid, a value of 10^3 reflects a lung concentration of 10^6. PSB would suffer from lack of sensitivity and it is unviable in 10% of authentic pneumonia. In patients with localized new infiltrates, PSB is the procedure of choice. There are two kinds of constraints: one must use a fiber-optic bronchoscope to direct the brush, and one must examine the sample within 1 h [39].

An alternative to the PSB is the Plugged Telescoping Catheter (PTC). Its practicality and its sensitivity should even be superior, and there should be no difference between results collected by directed and non-directed PTC [37]. This fact must be confirmed by a larger number of series. The modification of a previous antibiotherapy or starting up a new antibiotherapy leads to a high risk of obtaining negative result of distal bacteriological samples.

Two types of protocols seem to be interesting:

The first consists, in clinically suspect patients, to carrying out only the BAL. Those patients who have a bronchopulmonary infection are immediately identified, thanks to the microscopic cell examination data, and the cultures of the alveolar lavage liquid are only realized in this sub-group. The second protocol consists in systematically carrying out a Wimberley brush sample just before BAL. Cytologic examination of the cells retrieved from the lavage liquid allows to start up or not immediately an antibiotherapy which can eventually be modified, according to the results of the brush cultures. Thus, one can avoid contamination of the lavage liquid by the flora colonizing the upper airway since only the brush sample is cultivated. The combination of the results of the two examinations whose technique differs permits a decrease in the risk of missing a veritable pulmonary infection.

Treatment

The treatment of pulmonary infections must be both preventive and curative.

The preventive treatment consists of:

1) *The use of all hygienic measures* aiming to limit exogenous contamination: disinfection of water outlets, regular cleaning, immediate disposal of soiled elements, hand washing by the staff, cleaning the stethoscope after each examination, changing of the proximal ringed join of the respirator, use of heating humidifiers [27], rigourous asepsis for any invasive actions.
2) *Oropharingeal decontamination:*
   The value of digestive decontamination has yet to be proved. Anti-gram-negative bacteria administration leads to a colonization with gram-positive bacteria. However, the use of sulfacrate rather than antacids and H_2 blockers appears to decrease the bacterial overgrowth in the upper portion of the gastro-intestinal tract and may influence the incidence of pulmonary infections in such patients [12]. Finally, the best prevention of digestive hemorrhage remains an adequate resuscitation together with an early feeding.
3) *The prevention and/or treatment of nosocomial sinusitis:*
   The use of orogastric rather than naso-gastric tubes, orotracheal intubation or carrying out a tracheostomy are needed for prevention [23]. When intubation is nasotracheal, one needs to confirm the possible sinusitis diagnosis by a scanography. In the case of a radiological certainty, it is recommended to carry out a trans-nasal puncture of the maxillary sinus under general anesthesia to drain and to wash daily with an aminoglucoside. The presence of a nasogastric tube leads to a maxillary sinusitis in more than 30% of cases.
4) *Intratracheal decontamination* for 2 weeks could be a good way to decrease the number of nosocomial pneumonia (polymyxin B). This has to be confirmed. Administering i.v. penicillin would allow to fight against the saprophyte flora of the oropharynx (streptococcus, corynebacteria, neisseria, anaerobics).
5) *The right choice of administered drugs:*
   - prophylactic use of antibiotics should be discouraged unless clearly indicated [1].
   - a well-suited antimicrobial treatment does not sterilize the burn wound, but maintains the microbial density below 10^5 organisms per gram of tissue, a level which even the immunocompromized burn patient can reasonably defend.

The advent of specific topical antimicrobial therapy, the use of more effective topics and well adapted systemic antibiotics together with early excision and grafting of the burn wound have dramatically decreased the frequency of pneumonia in burn patients resulting from direct hematogenous dissemination from the wound to the lungs [10].

The use of corticosteroids must remain exceptional. On the other hand, therapy with non-steroidal anti-inflammatory drugs to inhibit production of prostaglandin compounds by the cyclooxygenase pathway initiated early after the burn injury could fully restore the bactericidal activity of neutrophils and have beneficial effects on cell-mediated immune responses [34].

Morever, the fact that the classical complement pathway is almost intact suggests that passive or active immunization could be useful by recruiting bactericidal, chemotactic, and opsonic activities and could help to avoid infectious complications. Finally, the preservation of a good nutritional status is an important aspect in the prophylactic treatment of pulmonary infections.

Curative treatment

Therapy for pulmonary infections is often dictated by the clinical setting. In practice, the clinician asks himself three questions: Is it necessary to treat? When to treat? How to treat?

Is it necessary to treat?

When a vital prognosis is involved, a rigid attitude is not justified and a minimum of arguments is enough, but it is necessary to begin rapidly the antibiotherapy. Serious cases are linked to pneumonia itself and to underlying pathology. The following situations justify the possible use of antibiotics:

1) Previous underlying pulmonary damage straight away creating a handicap.
2) Hypoxemiant pneumopathy, extensive or rapidly spreading.
3) Pneumopathy responsible for a state of shock for multi-organ failure and/or a septicemic syndrome.
4) Severe immunodeficiency (aplasia, long-term steroid treatment, AIDS).
5) Presumption of a bacterial etiology based on the local ecology (for instance, the presence of a virulent strain).

The most usual clinical signs are: Infectious syndrome (fever or hypothermia); purulent tracheal secretions; radiological infiltrate.

If there are previous anomalies (ARDS, pre-existing pneumopathy) rendering all precise radiological semiology illusive, one will need to be satisfied with modification of the images and, even with a septic state non easily explicable by an extra-pulmonary pathology. Bacteriological investigations remain indispensable, but a well thought-out approach concerning the choice and indication of the antibiotherapy is justified [33]. Indeed, Kreger has shown that half of the deaths during BGN septicemia occur in the first 24 h, and this is a good argument for urgency of an effective therapy. In a group of patients treated with aminoglycosides, Moore finds a 21 % mortality rate when the initial peak is sub-therapeutic versus 2.4 % when it is imme-

diately elevated. If the state of the patient is not a cause for worry, the intention to treat relies on the same clinical and radiological arguments, but it is at that time desirable to postpone antibiotherapy by 24 h. This interval allows:
 1) to try to eliminate an eventually non-infectious pathology (edema, atelectasis, infarction);
 2) to refine the diagnosis of pneumonia by specific and sensible explorations.

Is it necessary to treat and when?

Finally, as Wolff suggests, one can separate situations necessitating an emergency treatment (I) from those in which it can be postponed (II).

An example can be shown from the therapeutic schema in use at the C. Bernard Hospital during a presumed nosocomial pneumopathy in intubated or tracheotomized patients [22] (see Tables 1 and 2).

How to treat?

Antibiotherapy for pneumonia remains difficult. Emergency situations and frequent initial lack of bacterial identification most often make the use of empiric antibiotherapy obligatory. The above aims to cover the maximum varieties of germs, bacterial resistances, rendering null and void the efficacy of antibiotics.

Predominant bacteria are gram-negative bacteria (*P. aeruginosa*, group of KES), *staph. aureus* [2]. One must be aware of the possibility of a polymicrobial etiology as well as necessity to take into account gram-positive cocci, not only *Staph. aureus methi. R*, but also *S. pneumoniae*.

Agents which can be used are well known:

- *Third generation cephalosporins* (3GC) Their stability to beta-lactamases gives them a wide activity spectrum for resistant gram bacteria to 1GC and 2 GC including the majority of *Pseudomonas* for ceftazidim cefoperazone, but they are inactive on *S. aureus methi-R*. Moreover, plasmidic resistances by cephalosporinases production are described for *Enterobacter* and *Klebsiella* [29].
- *Monobactams*: They have a limited spectrum for gram-negative bacteria. Inactivation by enterobacteria producing cephalosporins is well known.
- *Carbapenems*: Imipenem has the widest spectrum, but *Cepacia* and *P. maltophila* are ordinary resistant.
- *Fluoroquinolones*: Very active on gram-negative bacteria, *S. aureus* and many *P. aeruginosa*; they are inactive on anaerobies and have a poor activity on *Streptococcus* (*S. pneumoniae*).
- *Aminosides*: They are an indispensable component of associations. Amikacin has the more stable activity on hospital bacteria [28].
- *Vancomycine and Teicoplamine*: Their activity on *Methy-R. staphilococci* is of the most interest.

The final question, mono- or bi-therapy?

The use of 3GC alone (monotherapy) leads to failure rate by emergence of resistant strains significantly greater than their association with an aminoglycoside.

Table 1. The patient is in a worrisome clinical situation:

He/she needs urgent antibiotherapy (ATB)

| Day 0, H. 0 | – Sample for direct examination (DE)
– PSB

Positive result of DE → directed ATB
Negative result of DE → wide spectrum ATB according to local flora

| Day 1, H. 24 | clinical, radiological re-evaluation

$PSB \geq 10^3$ CFU/ml → continuation and then adaptation of ATB

$PSB < 10^3$/ml
- if ≥ 3 days previous ATB → continuation of ATB
- no previous ATB or <3 days ATB → continuation of ATB depending on the context (extrapulmonary sepsis? non-infectious pneumopathy?)

Table 2. The patient is in a non-worrisome clinical situation

Antibiotherapy (ATB) is deferred.
Treatment is symptomatic.

| Day 0, H. 0 | – sample for direct examination (DE). Results to be taken into account if the situation becomes worrisome
– PSB

| Day 1, H. 24 | clinical and radiological re-evaluation

The therapy will depend on the results of PSB:

1 – persistent infiltrate + $PSB \geq 10^3$ cfu/ml → ATB
2 – ✓✓ infiltrate + $PSB < 10^3$ /ml → no ATB
3 – ✓✓ infiltrate + $PSB \geq 10^3$ /ml → no ATB but regular clinical and radiological re-evaluation

4 – persistent infiltrate + $PSB < 10$ /ml

no ATB or ATB less than 3 days
- no ATB
- or
- stop ATB

ATB before ≥ 3 days
- stop ATB
- 2nd PSB after 24 h

Fluoroquinolones also provoke an emergence of resistance. Imipenem induces persistent colonization or emergence of resistant strains of pseudomonas and staphylococcus [24].

The basic principle for empiric antibiotherapy of pulmonary infections and, particularly, of pneumonia is bi-therapy. The analysis of the results of numerous multicentric French studies reveals a recovery rate significantly higher when the bacteria is sensitive to both antibiotics.

Empiric antibiotherapy for nosocomial pneumonia is realistic only if one takes into account bacterial ecology of each burn patient (eventually of the burn unit) and the spectrum of association. Whenever possible, the use of specific antibiotics on pre-diagnosed bacteria leads to a greater success rate in the treatment of pulmonary infections and particularly pneumonia.

References

1. Aerdts JA, Van Dalem R, Clasener AL (1991) Antibiotic prophylaxis of respiratory tract infection in mechanically ventilated patients. Chest 100:783–791
2. Bates JH (1989) Microbial etiology of pneumonia. Chest 9 (suppl.):194S–199S
3. Benoni G, Cuzzolin L, Bertrand C (1987) Imipenem kinetics in serum, lung tissue and pericardial fluid in patients undergoing thoracotomy. J of antimicr Chemoth 20:725–728
4. Borderon E, Leprince A, Gueveler C, Borderon JC (1981) Valeur des examens bactériologiques des sécrétions trachéales; comparaison avec les résultats des biopsies pulmonaires. Rev Fr Mal Resp 9:229–239
5. Chastre J, Fagon JY, Soler P (1988) Diagnosis of nosocomial bacterial pneumonia in intubated patients undergoing ventilation: comparison of the usefulness of bronchoalveolar lavage and the protected specimen brush. Am J Med 85:499–509
6. Chastre J, Fagon JY, Soler P (1989) Quantification of BAL cells containing intracellular bacteria rapidly identifies ventilated patients with nosocomial pneumonia. Chest 95:1905–1925
7. Craven DE, Daschner FD (1989) Nosocomial pneumonia in the intubated patient: role of gastric colinization. Eur J clin microbiol Infect Dis 8:40–80
8. Craven DE, Kunches LM, Kilinsky V (1986) Risk factors for pneumonia anf fatality in patients receiving continuous mechanical ventilation. Am Rev Respir Dis 133:792–796
9. Cross AS, Roup B (1981) Role of respiratory assistance devices in endemic nosocomial pneumonia. Am J of Med 70:681–685
10. Demling RH (1983) Improved survival after massive burns. J Trauma 23:179–184
11. Demling RH, Wong C, Jin LJ (1985) Early lung dysfunction after major burns: role of edema and vaso-active mediators. J of Trauma 10:959–966
12. Driks MR, Craven DE, Celli BR (1987) Nosocomial pneumonia in intubated patients giving sucralfate as compared with antacids or histamine type 2 blockers. N Engl J Med 10:355–357
13. Fagon JY, Chastres J, Hance AJ (1988) Detection of nosocomial lung infection in ventilated patients. Use of a protected specimen brush and quantitative cultures techniques in 147 patients. Am rev Respir Dis 138:110–116
14. Federle MP, Mark AS, Guillaumin ES (1986) CT of subpulmonic pleural effusions and atelectasis: criteria for differentiation from subphrenic fluid. AJR 146:685–689
15. Garibaldi RA, Britt MR, Coleman MC (1981) Risk factors for post-operative pneumonias. Am J Med 70:677–683
16. Herndon DN, Barrow RE, Traber DL (1987) Extravascular lung water changes following smoke inhalation and massive burn injury. Surgery 102:341–348
17. Herndon DN, Langer F, Thompson P (1987) Pulmonary injury in burned patients. Surg Clin North Am 67:31–46
18. Herndon DN, Langer F, Thompson P (1987) Pulmonary injury in burned patients. Surg Clin North Am 67:31

19. Herndon DN, Thompson PB, Linares HA (1986) Postgraduate course: respiratory injury – Part I. J Burn Care Rehab 7:184–191
20. Hubert Ch, Carette MF, Lebreton C, Bonnel D (1986) L'angiographie pulmonaire numérique. Etude comparée de deux techniques. Asservissement à l'électrocardiogramme versus trois images par seconde. J Radiol 67:377–379
21. Jin LJ, Lalonde C, Demling RH (1986) Lung dysfunction after thermal injury in relation to prostanoid and oxygen radical release. J Appl Physiol 61:103–110
22. Kahn RJ, Arich Ch, Baron D, Gutmann L (1990) Diagnostic des pneumopathies nosocomiales en réanimation. V. conference de concensus. Réan Soins Intens Méd Urg, 6, no 2, 91–124
23. Kerver AJ, Rommes JH, Mevissen-Verhage EAE (1988) Prevention of colonization and infection in critically ill patients. A prospective randomized study. Critical Care Med 16:1087–1093
24. La Force FM (1989) Systemic antimicrobial therapy of nosocomial pneumonia: monotherapy versus combination therapy. Eur J Clin Microbiol Infect Dis 8:61–68
25. Lambert RS, Vereen LE, George RB (1989) Comparison of tracheal aspirates and protected brush catheter specimens for identifying pathogenic bacteria in mechanically ventilated patients. Am J Med Sci 297:377–382
26. Maki DG (1989) Risk factors for nosocomial infection in intensive care: devices VS nature and goals for the next decade. Arch Intern Med 149:30–35
27. Misset B, Escudier B, Rivara D (1991) Heat and moisture exchanger vs. heated humidifier during long-term mechanical ventilation. Chest 100:160–163
28. Moore RD, Smith CR, Lietman PS (1984) Association of aminoglycoside plasma levels with therapeutic outcome in gram-negative pneumonia. Am J Med 77:657–662
29. Mouton Y, Deboscker Y, Beuscart C (1985) Third generation cephalosporins in combination with aminoglycosides or in monotherapy for life-threatening infections in an intensive care unit; in 25th ICAAC Minneapolis. Abstract no 958
30. Musset D, Rosso J, Petitprez P (1988) Acute pulmonary embolism: diagnostic value of digital subtraction angiography. Radiology 166:455–459
31. Peitzman AB, Shires GT, Teixidor HS (1989) Smoke inhalation injury: evaluation of radiographic manifestations and pulmonary dysfunction. J of Trauma 29:1232–1239
32. Rello J, Quintana E, Ausina V (1991) Incidence, etiology and outcome of nosocomial pneumonia in mechanically ventilated patient. Chest 100:439–442
33. Scheld WM, Mandell GL (1991) Nosocomial pneumonia: pathogenesis and recent advances in diagnosis and therapy. Rev Infect Dis Suppl 9:S743–751
34. Shinozawa Y, Hales CA, Jung W (1986) Ibuprofen prevents synthetic smoke-induced pulmonary edema. Am Rev Respir Dis 134:1145–1151
35. Shirani Khan Z, Pruitt BA, Mason AD (1987) The influence of inhalation injury and pneumonia on burn mortality. Ann Surg 205:82–87
36. Singer C, Armstrong D, Rosen PP, Waltzer PD, Yu R (1979) Diffuse pulmonary infiltrates in immunocompromised patients – prospective study of 80 cases. Am J Med 66:110–120
37. Torres A, De la Bellacasa JP, Rodriguez-Roisin T (1988) Diagnostic value of telescoping flugged catheters in mechanically ventilated patients with bacterial pneumonia using Metras catheter. Am Rev Respir Dis 138:117–120
38. Wiener MD, Garay SM, Leitman BS (1991) Imaging of the intensive care unit patient. Clinics in Chest Medicine 12:169–196
39. Wimberley N, Faling LJ, Bartlett JG (1979) A fiberoptic bronchoscopy technique to obtain uncontaminated lower airway secretions for bacterial culture. Am Rev Respir Dis 119:337–343
40. Zikria B, Ferrer J, Floch H (1972) The chemical factors contributing to pulmonary damage in smoke poisoning. Surgery 71:704–709

Address:
Dr. J Guilbaud
Hôpital d'Instruction des Armées Percy
101, Avenue Henri Barbusse
92141 Clamart
France

Die Beatmungstherapie beim Brandverletzten – Komplikationen und Outcome

R. Stuttmann

Abteilung für Anaesthesiologie, Kliniken der Stadt Köln, Krankenhaus Merheim, Köln

Die Bedeutung der Rauchgasinhalation bei einem Verbrennungstrauma ist schon in der ersten Hälfte des Jahrhunderts beschrieben worden. Eine Schädigung der Lunge durch die Inhalation von Rauchgasen verlängert die Behandlungsdauer, verschlechtert die Prognose eines Brandopfers und kann die alleinige Todesursache sein [1, 15, 20, 29, 33]. Eine große Zahl toxischer Produkte werden bei einem Brand freigesetzt [21]. Die pathophysiologischen Veränderungen der Lunge nach einer Rauchgasinhalation sind weitgehend aufgeklärt [6, 32]. Als diagnostisches Verfahren ist die fiberoptische Bronchoskopie geeignet, einen Inhalationsschaden zu erkennen. An der anatomischen Grenze der Stimmbänder wird der Inhalationsschaden der oberen Luftwege von einem Schaden des Tracheobronchialbaumes abgegrenzt [5, 12, 18]. Eine parenchymatöse Schädigung kann fiberoptisch nicht erkannt werden. Als Zeichen einer funktionellen Schädigung der Lungen kann nach einer Rauchgasinhalation eine Hypoxie eintreten [8, 14], der eine prognostische Bedeutung beigemessen wird [27, 34]. Bei einer respiratorischen Insuffizienz ist der Wert einer maschinellen Beatmung mit einem kontinuierlichen positiven Atemwegsdruck unbestritten [7, 9]. Wenig ist darüber bekannt, in welchem Ausmaß ein schlechter physiologischer Status eines Schwerbrandverletzten seine respiratorische Insuffizienz unterhält, zu einer Abhängigkeit von dem Respirator führt und die Letalität erhöht. Deshalb wurde prospektiv die Bedeutung des physiologischen Status des Patienten auf die Lungenfunktion und die Sterblichkeit untersucht.

Patienten und Methodik

Von Januar 1986 bis November 1991 wurden 193 brandverletzte Patienten, die länger als 48 Stunden beatmet werden mußten, in die Untersuchung aufgenommen. Es wurden folgende Basisdaten untersucht: das Alter, das Geschlecht, die verbrannte Körperoberfläche (VKO), der Anteil der drittgradig verbrannten Haut, der Schweregrad eines Inhalationstraumas, der „Abbreviated Burn Severity Index" (ABSI) als Verbrennungsscore [30], die Beatmungsdauer und die Sterblichkeit. Der Allgemeinzustand der Patienten wurde täglich durch Verlaufsparameter quantitativ erfaßt. Es wurden Störungen der Funktion eines Organs, klinische Diagnosen und ein erhöhter therapeutischer Aufwand als Variablen definiert. Grenzen für Funktionsstörungen waren z. B. ein systolischer arterieller Druck <90 mmHg oder ein Bilirubin >5 mg/dl. Ein erhöhter therapeutischer Aufwand war z. B. ein Dialyseverfahren. Abdominelle Störungen wurden als klinische Diagnosen wie z. B. „Peritonitis" oder „Ileus" erfaßt. Metabolische Störungen waren Elektrolyt- oder Blutzuckerentgleisungen, Störungen des Säure-Basen-Haushaltes oder eine Laktatämie. Mit der Hilfe einer Liste der zu prüfenden Parameter wurde täglich nach Veränderungen der Funktion des Kreislaufs, der Nieren, der Leber, des Stoffwechsels, des Abdomens und nach Sepsiszeichen gesucht. Alle Störungen wurden als gleichberechtigte, qualitative Variablen (0 = Bedingung nicht erfüllt oder 1 = Bedingung erfüllt) in einem Datenbanksystem (D-BASE IV, Ashton-Tate®) erfaßt (Mehrfachnennungen in einem Organgebiet waren möglich). Die Basisdaten der Patienten wurden als numerische Variable protokolliert.

Diesen extrapulmonalen Störungen wurden täglich die Lungenfunktionsparameter gegenübergestellt. Als numerischer Parameter der Lungenfunktion wurde der Gasaustausch mit dem alveolo-arteriellen Sauerstoffquotienten bewertet ($AARO_2$ = $PalvO_2 - PaO_2/PalvO_2$; theoretischer Bereich von 0–1, Normalbereich <0,4) [2]. Die Lungendehnbarkeit wurde als statische Compliance aus dem Tidalvolumen und dem Atemwegsdruck errechnet. Als Komplikationen der Langzeitbeatmung wurden als klinische Diagnosen Pneumonien und ein ARDS ebenfalls als jeweils eine qualitative Variable in der Datenbank erfaßt.

Um Einflüsse durch unterschiedliche Beatmungsformen auszuschließen, wurden die Patienten standardisiert nach einem adaptiven Schema volumenkontrolliert normoventiliert. Ausgehend von einer Grundeinstellung (TV ≤ 10 ml/kgKG, AF ≤ 10/min, FiO_2 ≤ 0,3) wurde der Beatmungsaufwand stufenweise gesteigert oder nach Verbesserung der Beatmungssituation wieder reduziert (Zielparameter: PaO_2 > 80 mmHg). Der Beatmungsmehraufwand betraf in zwei Stufen die Ventilation [1) TV ≤ 13 ml/kgKG, AF ≤ 13/min. 2) TV > 13 ml/kgKG, AF > 13/min] und in vier Stufen die Oxygenation [Stufe 1) FiO_2 ≤ 0,4, PEEP ≤ 5 cm H_2O. Stufe 2) I : E = 1 : 1. Stufe 3) bester PEEP. Stufe 4) I : E = 2 : 1, FiO_2 > 0,4, ggf. hämodynamisches Monitoring zur Optimierung der Kreislaufsituation].

Die primäre Versorgung des schwerverbrannten Patienten war ebenfalls standardisiert. Nach der Aufnahme der Patienten in die Klinik wurden nach einem Reinigungsbad die Verbrennungswunden oberflächlich nekrosektomiert. Danach wurde die Fläche der verbrannten Haut abgeschätzt. Die Tiefe der Verbrennung der Haut wurde klinisch beurteilt, und es wurden tief dermale (2 b) von drittgradig verbrannten Arealen unterschieden. Wenn anamnestisch z. B. aufgrund einer Verbrennung im geschlossenen Raum, bei Verbrennungen des Gesichtes oder bei Störungen der Atmung der Verdacht eines Inhalationstraumas bestand, wurden die Patienten bronchoskopiert. Diagnostische Kriterien für einen Inhalationsschaden waren Schleimhautrötung, Schleimhautschwellung, Bildung von Pseudomembranen, Rußauflagerungen und Schleimhautnekrosen. Zur Überwachung der Lungenfunktion wurden mindestens 4stündlich Blutgase analysiert und der alveolo-arterielle Sauerstoffquotient berechnet. 24 Stunden nach dem Verbrennungsunfall wurde das arithmetische Mittel errechnet. Nach dem bronchoskopischen Befund und dem Mittelwert des alveolo-arteriellen Sauerstoffquotienten wurde 24 Stunden nach der Verbrennung das Inhalationstrauma in drei Schweregrade eingeteilt. Als erstgradiges Inhalationstrauma wird klassifiziert, wenn der Verdacht eines Inhalationsschadens z. B. bei Verbrennungen des Gesichtes besteht, aber weder der Luftweg geschädigt noch der Gasaustausch gestört sind. Ein zweitgradiges Inhalationstrauma liegt vor, wenn bronchoskopisch eine Schädigung des Bronchialbaums erkannt wird, der Gasaustausch der Lunge aber weitgehend ungestört ist (Mittelwert des alveolo-arteriellen Sauerstoffquotienten der ersten 24 Stunden nach dem Trauma ≤ 0,4). Es liegt ein drittgradiges Inhalationstrauma vor, wenn der Luftweg geschädigt und zusätzlich auch der Gasaustausch der Lunge gestört sind (Mittelwert des alveolo-arteriellen Sauerstoffquotienten der ersten 24 Stunden nach dem Trauma > 0,4) [26]. Nach der

Feststellung des Schweregrades des Inhalationsschadens wurde das gesamte Verbrennungstrauma nach dem ABSI klassifiziert.

Hauptzielkriterium der Untersuchung war die Sterblichkeit. Es wurde der Einfluß des Alters, des Geschlechts, des Inhalationstraumas und des physiologischen Zustandes auf die Sterblichkeit untersucht. Folgende Patientengruppen wurden verglichen: 1) Patienten, die jünger als 60 Jahre waren mit Patienten, die 60 Jahre oder älter waren; 2) weibliche Patienten mit männlichen Patienten; 3) Patienten ohne Inhalationstrauma mit Patienten mit einem zweitgradigen oder einem drittgradigen Inhalationstrauma. Zur Beschreibung des physiologischen Grundzustandes der Patienten wurde täglich die Summe der extrapulmonalen Störungen, der alveoloarterielle Sauerstoffquotient, die Lungendehnbarkeit (Compliance), die Häufigkeit von Pneumonien und eines ARDS errechnet. Untersucht wurde ein Zeitraum von 42 Tagen. Der Tag der Extubation bzw. des Ablebens der Patienten war der erste Untersuchungstag. Von diesem Zeitpunkt an wurde der physiologische Zustand der Patienten 42 Beatmungstage zurück verfolgt. Es wurden überlebende mit verstorbenen Patienten verglichen.

Statistik

Die Daten werden als Mittelwert mit Standardabweichung dargestellt.

Ergebnisse

Basisdaten

Von den Patienten überlebten 100 und 93 verstarben. Die Verstorbenen waren älter, hatten eine größere Verbrennungsfläche und einen höheren Verbrennungsscore. Das Geschlecht von 50 Patienten war weiblich und von 143 Patienten männlich. Es verstarben von den 50 weiblichen Patienten 36 (72%) und von den 143 männlichen Patienten 55 (38%). Das Alter und der Verbrennungsscore der verstorbenen weiblichen Patienten war höher (58 Jahre, 10,4 Scorepunkte) als bei männlichen Patienten (40 Jahre, 9,4 Scorepunkte) (Tabelle 1).

Tabelle 1. Basisdaten des Untersuchungskollektivs

	Anzahl	Alter Jahre	VKO %	Score Punkte	Beatmung Tage
Anzahl gesamt	193	40 (19)	36 (22)	7,3 (3,6)	23 (23)
Überlebende	100	35 (15)	28 (16)	6,3 (2,8)	25 (24)
Verstorbene	93	47 (21)	44 (26)	8,7 (3,9)	21 (21)
Überlebende Männer	88	34 (15)	28 (15)	6,9 (1,8)	27 (23)
Überlebende Frauen	14	36 (16)	29 (15)	7,9 (1,6)	18 (27)
Verstorbene Männer	55	40 (17)	47 (27)	9,4 (2,6)	23 (24)
Verstorbene Frauen	36	58 (21)	41 (25)	10,4 (2,5)	19 (15)

Daten als Mittelwerte mit Standardabweichung in Klammern. Der Unterschied in der Beatmungsdauer zwischen männlichen und weiblichen Patienten ist signifikant (t-test, $p < 0,05$).

Tabelle 2a. Basisdaten der Patienten jünger als 60 Jahre

	Anzahl	Alter Jahre	VKO %	Score Punkte
Gesamt	162	34 (13)	38 (23)	8,1 (2,5)
Männer	130	33 (12)	37 (22)	7,8 (2,4)
Frauen	32	37 (12)	41 (24)	9,3 (2,6)
Überlebende Männer	83	32 (12)	30 (15)	6,9 (1,8)
Überlebende Frauen	14	32 (12)	29 (15)	7,9 (1,6)
Verstorbene Männer	47	34 (13)	51 (26)	9,3 (2,5)
Verstorbene Frauen	18	40 (12)	48 (26)	10,2 (2,8)

Daten als Mittelwerte mit Standardabweichung in Klammern. Weibliche Patienten haben eine höhere Sterblichkeit.

Tabelle 2b. Basisdaten der Patienten älter als 60 Jahre

	Anzahl	Alter Jahre	VKO %	Score Punkte
Gesamt	31	73 (9)	32 (21)	9,7 (2,7)
Männer	12	69 (9)	31 (22)	8,8 (2,9)
Frauen	19	76 (6)	32 (20)	10,5 (2,3)
Überlebende Männer	5	70 (11)	19 (9)	7,4 (1,1)
Überlebende Frauen	0	–	–	–
Verstorbene Männer	7	69 (10)	39 (25)	9,7 (3,3)
Verstorbene Frauen	19	76 (6)	32 (20)	10,5 (2,3)

Daten als Mittelwerte mit Standardabweichung in Klammern. Alle weiblichen Patienten sind verstorben im Vergleich zu 42% der männlichen Patienten. Die Verletzungsschwere ist vergleichbar.

Einflüsse durch das Alter der Patienten

Es waren 162 Patienten jünger als 60 Jahre. Davon waren 32 Patienten weiblich und 130 Patienten männlich. Der Verbrennungsscore weiblicher Patienten war höher (9,3 versus 7,8 Scorepunkte) als bei männlichen Patienten. Es verstarben 18 weibliche (56%) und 47 männliche (36%) Patienten. Weitere Daten sind in der Tabelle 2a enthalten.

31 Patienten waren 60 Jahre alt oder älter. Aus diesem Kollektiv war der Verbrennungsscore der 19 weiblichen Patienten höher (10,5 Scorepunkte) als bei den 12 männlichen Patienten (8,8 Scorepunkte). Alle weiblichen Patienten verstarben im Vergleich zu 7 (58%) der 12 männlichen Brandopfer (Tabelle 2b).

Einflüsse durch ein Inhalationstrauma

Von den 193 Patienten hatten 44 ein Inhalationstrauma zweiten Grades und 84 ein Inhalationstrauma dritten Grades. Bei 65 Patienten lag kein Inhalationstrauma als primärer Beatmungsgrund vor. Die Sterblichkeit der Patienten mit einem zweitgra-

Tabelle 3. Basisdaten der Patienten mit einem Inhalationstrauma II. Grades, III. Grades und einer Beatmung aufgrund anderer Ursachen (kein Inhalationstrauma)

	Anzahl	Alter Jahre	VKO %	Score Punkte	Beatmung Tage
Kein Inhalationstrauma	65	40 (23)	36 (23)	7,7 (2,4)	18 (18
Verstorbene	28	48 (27)	47 (28)	9,2 (2,5)	19 (16)
Überlebende	37	35 (18)	29 (15)	6,8 (1,7)	16 (19)
Inhalationstrauma II. Grades	44	33 (15)	39 (22)	8,3 (2,8)	20 (20)
Verstorbene	14	43 (20)	55 (26)	11,0 (2,7)	20 (17)
Überlebende	30	28 (9)	32 (13)	7,1 (1,8)	21 (22)
Inhalationstrauma III. Grades	84	43 (15)	37 (22)	8,7 (2,6)	29 (26)
Verstorbene	51	46 (16)	43 (24)	9,7 (2,6)	23 (24)
Überlebende	33	39 (13)	28 (15)	7,4 (1,8)	39 (24)

Daten als Mittelwerte mit Standardabweichung in Klammern. Die Sterblichkeit und die Beatmungsdauer nehmen mit ansteigendem Schweregrad des Inhalationstraumas zu.

digen Inhalationstrauma (14 Patienten/32%) war geringer im Vergleich zu Patienten mit einem drittgradigen Inhalationstrauma (51 Patienten/61%) und im Vergleich zu Patienten ohne ein Inhalationstrauma (28 Patienten/43%). Das Alter und der Verbrennungsscore war bei den Verstorbenen deutlich höher als bei Überlebenden. Die Beatmung dauerte bei einem drittgradigen Inhalationstrauma länger als bei einem zweitgradigen (Tabelle 3).

Extrapulmonale Organstörungen

Alle Organe

Die täglich errechnete Summe aller extrapulmonalen physiologischen Störungen war bei den überlebenden Patienten an allen Untersuchungstagen niedriger als bei den Verstorbenen. Die extrapulmonalen Störungen nahmen bei den Überlebenden langsam bis zum Tage der Extubation ab. Im Vergleich wurde eine Zunahme bei den Verstorbenen beobachtet, besonders deutlich 14 Tage vor dem Tod. Überlebende Patienten hatten weniger extrapulmonale Störungen als Patienten, die verstarben. Es wurden bei den Überlebenden vorübergehend mehr als zwei bis maximal drei extrapulmonale Störungen beobachtet im Vergleich zu mehr als drei extrapulmonalen Störungen bei den Verstorbenen (Abb. 1).

Die häufigsten Nennungen waren Sepsisparameter, gefolgt von Störungen der Kreislauffunktion, des Metabolismus, der Nieren- und der Leberfunktion.

Sepsisparameter

Die Zahl der Sepsiszeichen nahm bei Überlebenden beginnend 12 Tage vor der Extubation stetig ab. Bei Verstorbenen wurde eine Zunahme der Sepsiskriterien bis zum Tode beobachtet (Abb. 2).

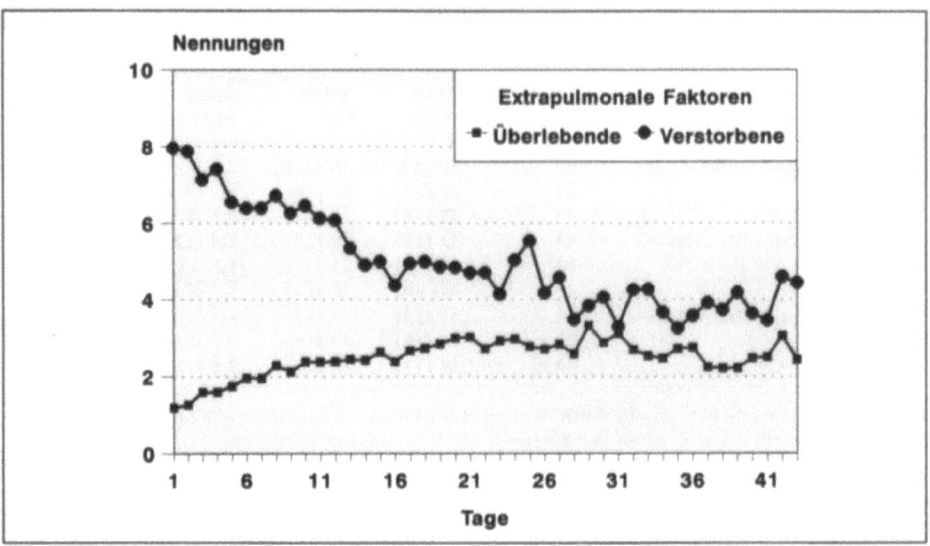

Abb. 1. Mittelwerte der Summe der nicht pulmonalen Organstörungen (Extrapulmonale Faktoren, maximal 54 Variablen) pro Patient. Tag 1 = Tag der Extubation (Gruppe der Überlebenden) bzw. Todestag (Gruppe der Verstorbenen). Tag 1–43 = Beatmungstage vor Extubation bzw. Exitus

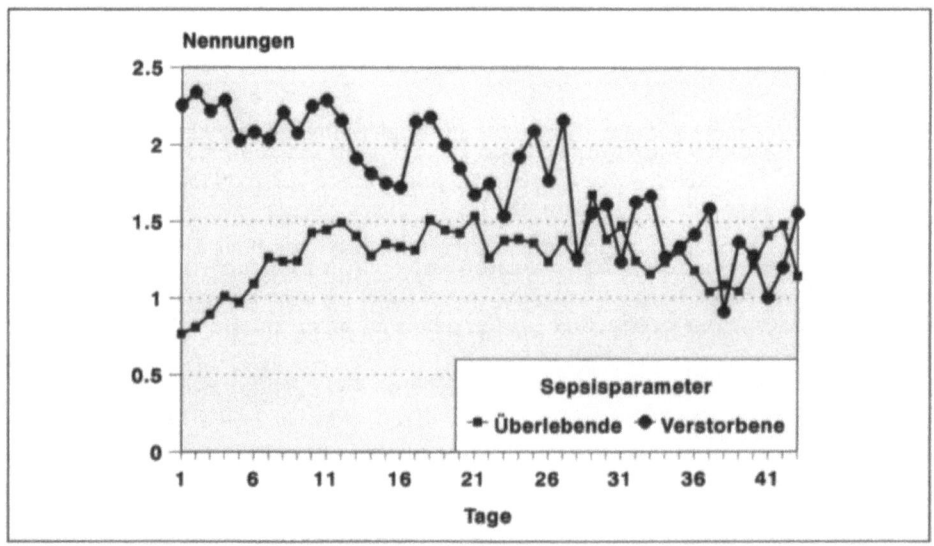

Abb. 2. Mittelwerte der Summe der Sepsisparameter (maximal 8) pro Patient. Tag 1 = Tag der Extubation (Gruppe der Überlebenden) bzw. Todestag (Gruppe der Verstorbenen). Tag 1–43 = Beatmungstage vor Extubation bzw. Exitus

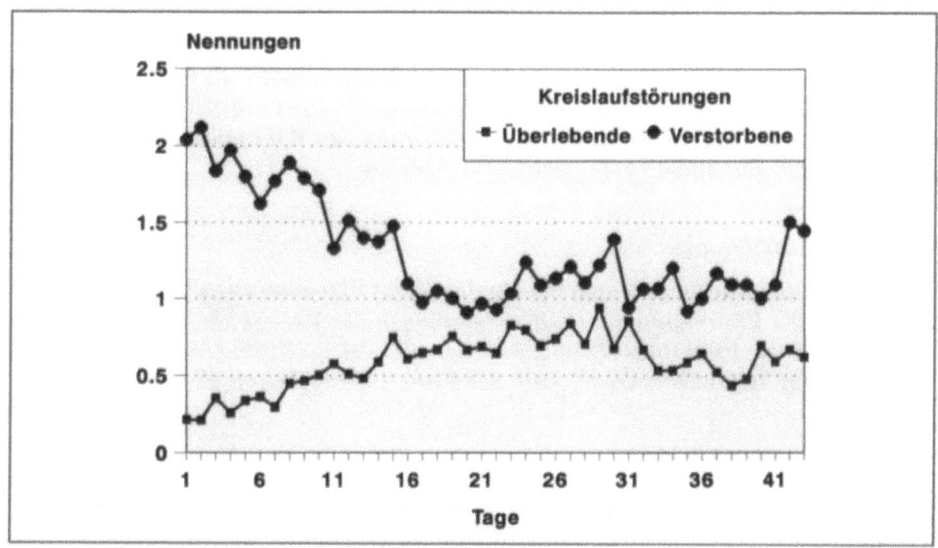

Abb. 3. Mittelwerte der Summe der Funktionsstörungen des Kreislaufs (maximal 9) pro Patient.
Tag 1 = Tag der Extubation (Gruppe der Überlebenden) bzw. Todestag (Gruppe der Verstorbenen).
Tag 1–43 = Beatmungstage vor Extubation bzw. Exitus

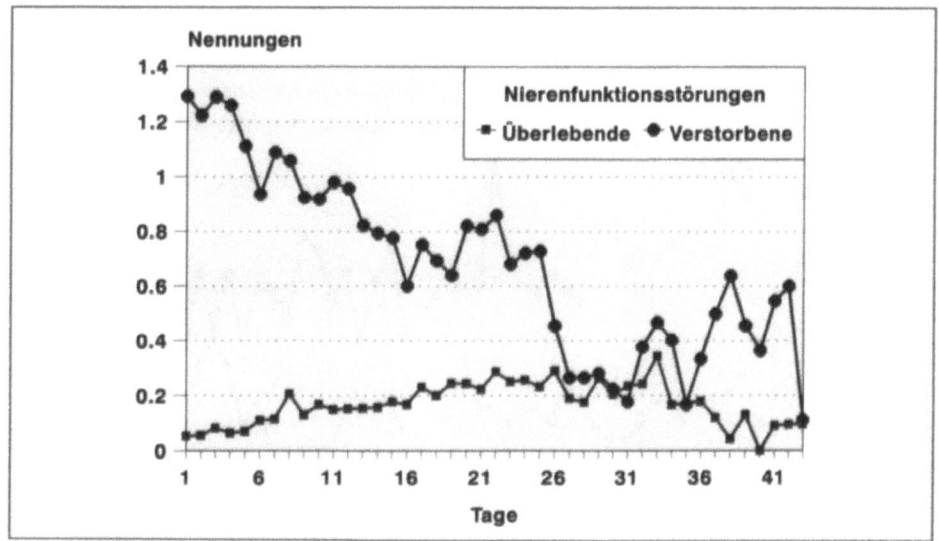

Abb. 4. Mittelwerte der Summe der Funktionsstörungen der Niere (maximal 8) pro Patient.
Tag 1 = Tag der Extubation (Gruppe der Überlebenden) bzw. Todestag (Gruppe der Verstorbenen).
Tag 1–43 = Beatmungstage vor Extubation bzw. Exitus

Kreislaufstörungen

Bei überlebenden Patienten waren Kreislaufstörungen seltener als bei verstorbenen Patienten. Die Zahl der Störungen nahm langsam bis zur Extubation ab. Die Verstorbenen hatten durchschnittlich ca. eine Störung des Kreislaufs mit einer deutlichen, stetigen Zunahme 16 Tage vor dem Ableben (Abb. 3).

Nierenfunktionsstörungen

Nierenfunktionsstörungen traten bei überlebenden Patienten zwischen dem 17. und 28. Tag vor der Extubation mit ca. 0,2 Nennungen pro Patient auf. Bis zur Extubation nahmen die Funktionsstörungen weiter ab. Bei verstorbenen Patienten stieg schon 28 Tage vor dem Tode die Zahl der Funktionsstörungen an (Abb. 4).

Leberfunktionsstörungen

Leberfunktionsstörungen waren bei überlebenden Patienten selten. Die Verstorbenen hatten ca. 3mal häufiger Leberfunktionsstörungen. Eine trendähnliche Zunahme der Störungen begann 30 Tage vor dem Ableben (Abb. 5).

Metabolische Störungen

Sowohl bei überlebenden Patienten als auch bei Verstorbenen waren metabolische Störungen bis zum 22. Tag selten; die Häufigkeit war in beiden Gruppen gleich.

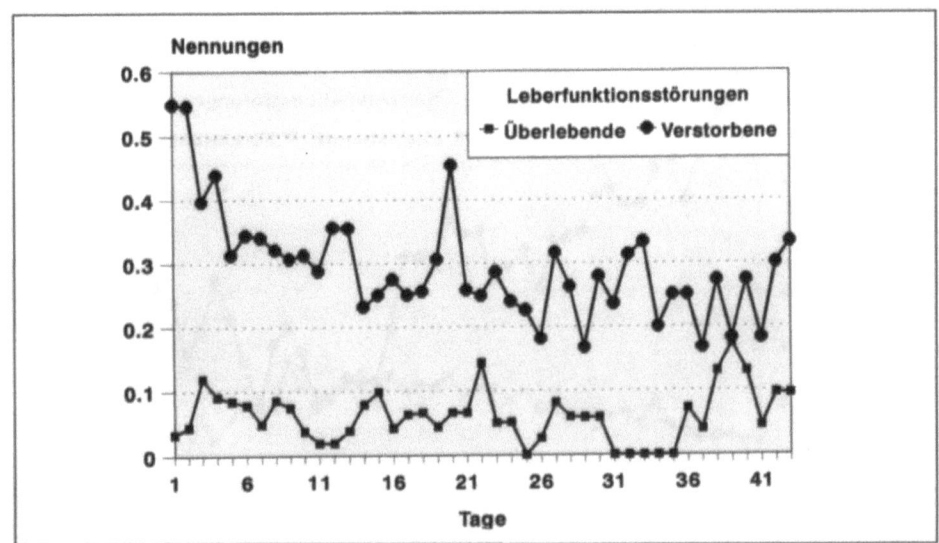

Abb. 5. Mittelwerte der Summe der Funktionsstörungen der Leber (maximal 5) pro Patient. Tag 1 = Tag der Extubation (Gruppe der Überlebenden) bzw. Todestag (Gruppe der Verstorbenen). Tag 1–43 = Beatmungstage vor Extubation bzw. Exitus

Beginnend 22 Tage vor dem Tode bzw. der Extubation nahmen die Störungen zu respektive ab (Abb. 6).

Pulmonale Störungen

Alveolo-arterieller Sauerstoffquotient

Der alveolo-arterielle Sauerstoffquotient war zwischen dem 38. und 42. Tag der Beobachtungsperiode zwischen den Gruppen nicht unterschiedlich. Am 38. und allen folgenden Tagen lag der Sauerstoffquotient der verstorbenen Patienten über den Werten der Überlebenden. Bei den Verstorbenen verschlechterte sich der Gasaustausch weiter mit einem deutlichen Anstieg des Quotienten in den letzten 2 Wochen vor dem Tod. Bei den Überlebenden fiel der Quotient langsam als Zeichen der Verbesserung der Lungenfunktion ab und erreichte 7 Tage vor der Extubation den Normalbereich (Abb. 7).

Lungendehnbarkeit

Die Lungendehnbarkeit war bei den überlebenden Patienten während des gesamten Beobachtungszeitraumes höher als bei den Verstorbenen. Bei diesen Patienten nahm die Lungendehnbarkeit bis zum Tode stetig ab (Abb. 8).

Pneumonien

Die Diagnose Pneumonie wurde bei überlebenden und verstorbenen Patienten mit gleicher Häufigkeit gestellt. Ausgehend von einer angedeuteten Zunahme der Inzi-

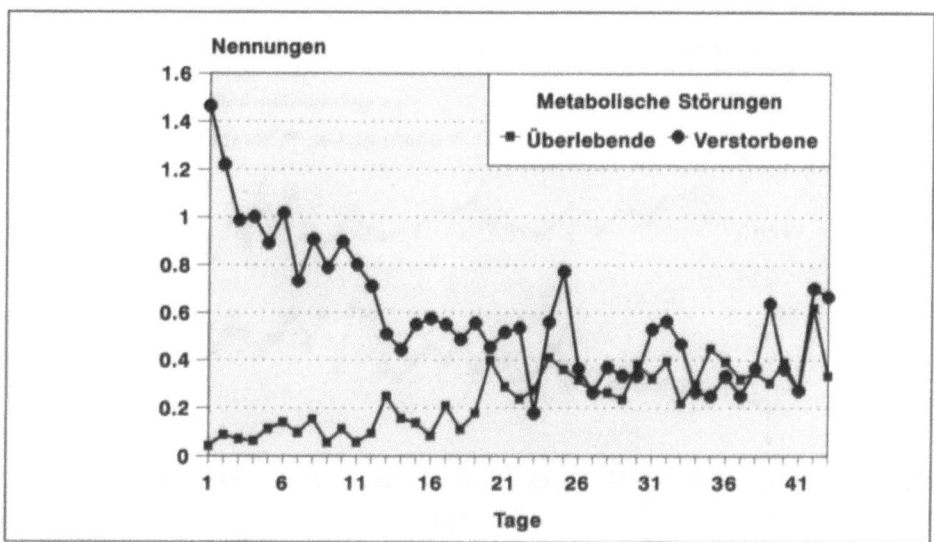

Abb. 6. Mittelwerte der Summe der metabolischen Störungen (maximal 5) pro Patient. Tag 1 = Tag der Extubation (Gruppe der Überlebenden) bzw. Todestag (Gruppe der Verstorbenen). Tag 1–43 = Beatmungstage vor Extubation bzw. Exitus

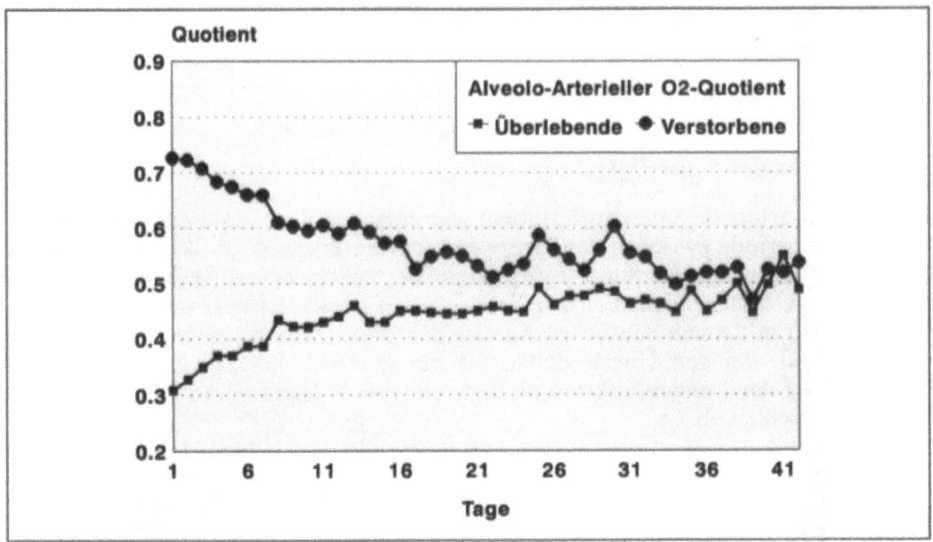

Abb. 7. Mittelwerte des alveolo-arteriellen Sauerstoffquotienten $PalvO_2-PartO_2/PalvO_2$. Tag 1 = Tag der Extubation (Gruppe der Überlebenden) bzw. Todestag (Gruppe der Verstorbenen). Tag 1–43 = Beatmungstage vor Extubation bzw. Exitus

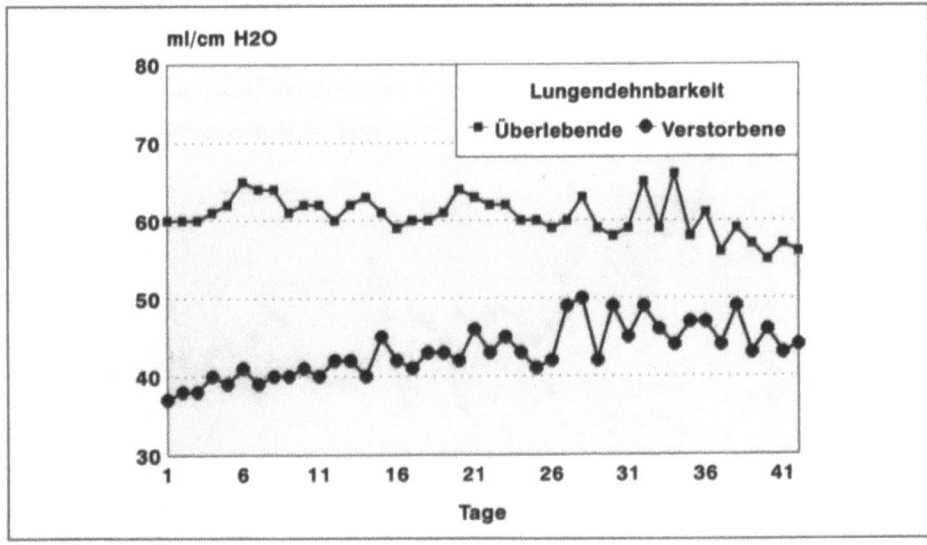

Abb. 8. Mittelwerte der Lungendehnbarkeit (ml/cmH$_2$O). Tag 1 = Tag der Extubation (Gruppe der Überlebenden) bzw. Todestag (Gruppe der Verstorbenen). Tag 1–43 = Beatmungstage vor Extubation bzw. Exitus

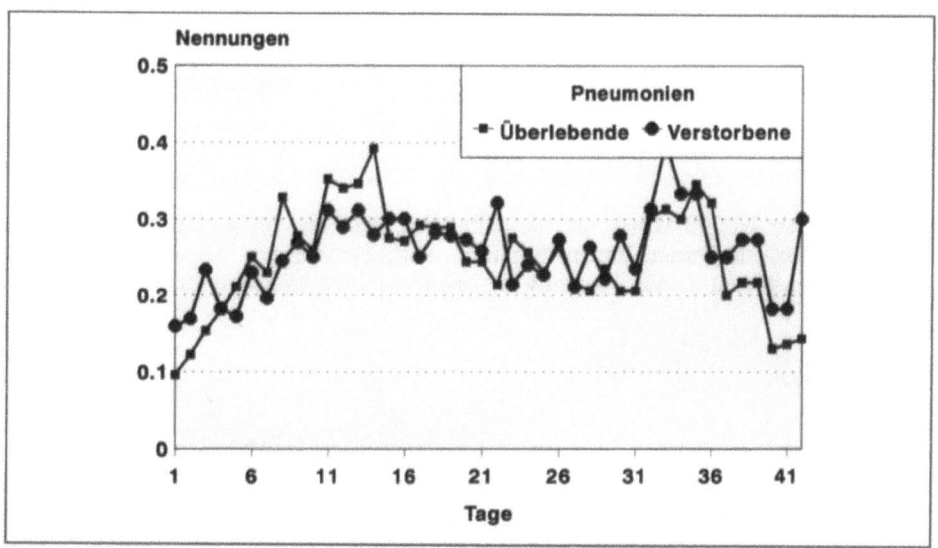

Abb. 9. Häufigkeit der Diagnose „Pneumonie" pro Patient und Beatmungstag. Tag 1 = Tag der Extubation (Gruppe der Überlebenden) bzw. Todestag (Gruppe der Verstorbenen). Tag 1–43 = Beatmungstage vor Extubation bzw. Exitus

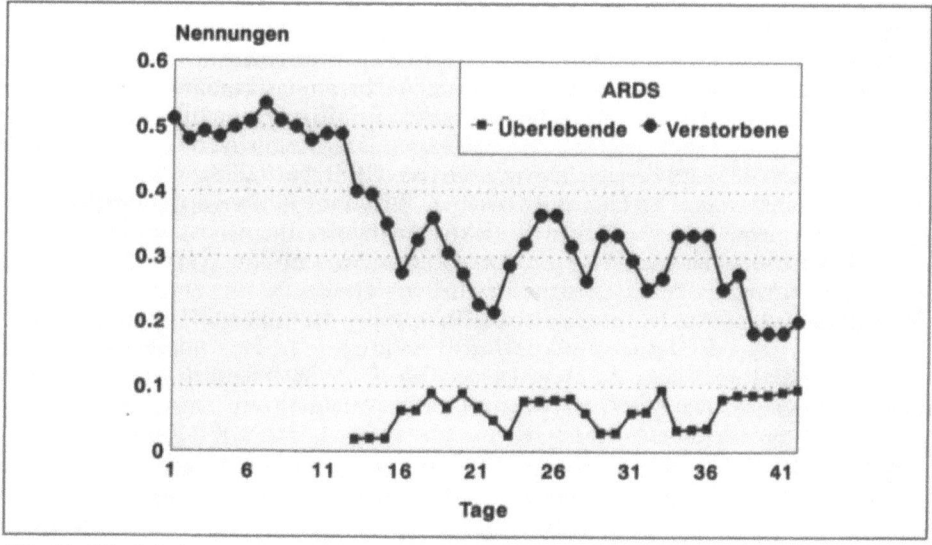

Abb. 10. Häufigkeiten der Diagnose „ARDS" pro Patient und Beatmungstag. Tag 1 = Tag der Extubation (Gruppe der Überlebenden) bzw. Todestag (Gruppe der Verstorbenen). Tag 1–43 = Beatmungstage vor Extubation bzw. Exitus

denz wurde in den letzten 2 Wochen der Beatmung sowohl bei überlebenden als auch bei verstorbenen Patienten eine Pneumonie mit abnehmender Häufigkeit diagnostiziert. Ein Unterschied zwischen den Gruppen war nicht erkennbar (Abb. 9).

ARDS

Die Diagnose ARDS wurde bei den überlebenden Patienten selten gestellt. Ein ARDS war bei den verstorbenen Patienten deutlich häufiger. Bei diesen Patienten wurde in den beiden letzten Wochen der Beatmung ein ARDS in ca. 50% der Fälle beobachtet.

Diskussion

Prognostische Indikatoren sind bei schwerverbrannten Patienten oft untersucht worden. Die originale Baux-Regel und die modifizierte Baux-Regel sind validierte Instrumente, um die Prognose eines Brandverletzten mit Hilfe der Variablen Alter und des Ausmaßes der verbrannten Körperoberfläche vorherzusagen [4, 25]. In einer großen Sammelstatistik über 10 Jahre von 1964 bis 1974 werden das weibliche Geschlecht und der Anteil der vollständig verbrannten Hautfläche als weitere Faktoren beschrieben, die die Sterblichkeit erhöhen [10]. Ein Inhalationstrauma wird in dem ABSI als zusätzliche prognostische Variable berücksichtigt, so daß der Score eine genauere Voraussage der Sterblichkeit zuläßt. Dieser Score wurde deshalb in der vorliegenden Erhebung benutzt, um die Schwere des Verbrennungstraumas und die Sterblichkeit zu untersuchen. Die Patientenkollektive für die Erhebung und Validierung des ABSI hatten eine Sterblichkeit von 15% bzw. 8%. Die verbrannte Körperoberfläche war in 81% kleiner als 30% [30, 31]. Die Patienten der vorliegenden Untersuchung wurden wegen einer respiratorischen Insuffizienz als Folge eines Inhalationstraumas oder einer Komplikation der Verbrennungskrankheit beatmet. Die Patienten haben als Ursache der respiratorischen Insuffizienz eine Inhalationsverletzung der Lunge oder eine septische Komplikation. Die Sterblichkeit des Gesamtkollektivs liegt mit 43% im Bereich der Angaben des ABSI. Nach diesem Score kann bei 8–9 Scorepunkten eine Sterblichkeit zwischen 30% und 50% erwartet werden. Verglichen mit einem uneinheitlichen Kollektiv beatmeter Intensivpatienten (>24 h) mit einer Sterblichkeit von 34%, sind diese Ergebnisse schlechter [11]. Die Patienten mit einem schweren Inhalationstrauma dritten Grades haben eine noch höhere Sterblichkeit von 60%. Die prognostische Bedeutung der initialen Hypoxie als Folge einer Schädigung der Lungenfunktion wird bestätigt [34]. Das Inhalationstrauma zweiten Grades ohne initiale Hypoxie hat bei einer Sterblichkeit von 32% eine bessere Prognose. Der ABSI der überlebenden Patienten mit einem Inhalationstrauma zweiten oder dritten Grades ist annähernd gleich. Der ABSI der verstorbenen Patienten mit einem Inhalationstrauma zweiten Grades ist um 1,6 Scorepunkte höher als bei Patienten mit einem drittgradigen Inhalationstrauma. Insgesamt ist die Prognose der Patienten mit einem zweitgradigen Inhalationstrauma besser im Vergleich zu Patienten mit einem drittgradigen Inhalationstrauma und zu Patienten ohne ein Inhalationstrauma, die als Folge einer Komplikation beatmet werden mußten. Das weibliche Geschlecht als negativer prognostischer Faktor wurde ebenfalls bestätigt. Unter

Berücksichtigung des Alters als weiteren Prognosefaktor ist die Sterblichkeit weiblicher Patienten unverändert höher als bei männlichen Patienten. Die hohe Sterblichkeit der über 60 Jahre alten Patienten kann die Folge schwerwiegender Vorerkrankungen sein. Eine beobachtete verzögerte Wundheilung begünstigt septische Komplikationen und kann dadurch die Prognose weiter verschlechtern [23, 28].

Die Darstellung der täglich erhobenen Verlaufsparameter zur Beschreibung des Allgemeinzustandes der Patienten unterscheidet sich in zwei wesentlichen Punkten von anderen Darstellungen. Erstens werden pulmonale Faktoren und extrapulmonale Faktoren getrennt dargestellt und zweitens sind die Datensätze der Patienten auf den Endpunkt der Respiratortherapie synchronisiert. Die Krankheitsverläufe werden jeweils beginnend am Tage der Extubation bzw. des Todes rückblickend verglichen. Im Beobachtungszeitraum haben die Verstorbenen immer eine höhere Anzahl extrapulmonaler Faktoren als die überlebenden Patienten. Sepsisparameter sind die häufigsten Faktoren gefolgt von Störungen des Kreislaufs und der Nierenfunktion. Der alveolo-arterielle Sauerstoffquotient und die Lungendehnbarkeit zeigen als pulmonale Faktoren gegenüber den extrapulmonalen Faktoren vergleichbare Verläufe. Ein ARDS ist bei überlebenden Patienten verglichen mit den Verstorbenen eine seltene Diagnose. Die Häufigkeit von Pneumonien unterscheidet sich nicht zwischen überlebenden und verstorbenen Patienten. Dieser Befund steht im Widerspruch zu einer Untersuchung, in der die Pneumonie ein Letalitätsfaktor ist, und die Inzidenz der Pneumonie mit dem Alter der Patienten und der verbrannten Körperoberfläche zunimmt [24].

Prognostische Indizes, die im Verlauf der Verbrennungskrankheit erhoben werden, sind z. B. biochemische Parameter [13], die Verbindung demographischer Daten mit Verlaufsparametern [19] und Sepsisparameter zur Beurteilung von therapeutischen Maßnahmen [17]. Bei verstorbenen Patienten ist die Zahl der untersuchten Faktoren im Verlauf ihrer Erkrankung signifikant höher als bei überlebenden Patienten. Die Patienten wurden entweder kontinuierlich bis zum 10. Behandlungstag [19] oder intermittierend bis zum 21. Behandlungstag untersucht [17]. Keine Erhebung erfaßt den gesamten Zeitraum der Behandlung. Die Prognose eines Schwerbrandverletzten verschlechtert sich mit einer verzögerten Wundheilung [22, 23]. Die Infektion einer nicht abgeheilten Verbrennungswunde kann eine systemische Reaktion mit den klinischen Zeichen eines septischen Syndroms hervorrufen [3, 16]. Sepsisparameter und die einer Sepsis folgenden Störungen des Kreislaufs, der Nierenfunktion, des Metabolismus und der Leberfunktion sind während des Beobachtungszeitraumes von 42 Tagen bei verstorbenen Patienten häufiger als bei Überlebenden. Diese Störungen werden als extrapulmonale Faktoren der Lungenfunktion gegenübergestellt. Die Verlaufsparameter der Lungenfunktion, der alveolo-arterielle Sauerstoffquotient und die Lungendehnbarkeit, verbessern sich ca. zwei Wochen vor der Extubation. Die Zahl extrapulmonaler Faktoren nimmt gleichzeitig ab. Bei den verstorbenen Patienten verschlechtern sich der alveolo-arterielle Sauerstoffquotient und die Lungendehnbarkeit. Bis zum Tode nimmt die Zahl extrapulmonaler Faktoren zu. Da der Unterschied zwischen überlebenden und verstorbenen Patienten mit der Dauer der Behandlung zunimmt, sind extrapulmonalen Faktoren, die im Krankheitsverlauf erworben werden, für die Prognose der Patienten von großer Bedeutung. Die Zahl extrapulmonaler Faktoren ist zwischen überlebenden und verstorbenen Patienten während des gesamten Beobachtungszeitraumes unterschiedlich. Der höhere Verletzungsscore der verstorbenen Patienten und die dadurch verstärkte pathologische Reaktion des Gesamtorganismus sind möglicherweise die Ursache.

Zusammenfassung und Schlußfolgerung

An 193 schwerverbrannten Patienten, die länger als 24 Stunden beatmet werden mußten, wurde die prognostische Bedeutung des Alters, des Geschlechts und des Inhalationstraumas geprüft. Die Prognose schwerverbrannter Patienten ist schlecht bei einem drittgradigen Inhalationstrauma, bei weiblichen Patienten und bei einem Alter über 60 Jahren. Die extrapulmonalen Faktoren und die pulmonalen Verlaufsparameter sind bei verstorbenen Patienten schon bei dem Beginn der Beatmung zahlreicher bzw. schlechter als bei überlebenden Patienten. Zwei Wochen vor dem Tod wird eine weitere Zunahme der Störungen beobachtet. Während des Krankheitsverlaufes erworbene neue extrapulmonale Faktoren verschlechtern die Prognose der beatmeten Patienten. Die von einer nicht heilenden Verbrennungswunde ausgehende Störung des Gesamtorganismus scheint für die Abhängigkeit von der Beatmung von entscheidender Bedeutung zu sein. Mit der Hilfe der Dokumentation von Verlaufsparametern muß ihre prognostische Bedeutung mit statistischen Methoden weiter untersucht werden.

Literatur

1. Aub JC, Pittman H, Brues AM (1943) The pulmonary complications: a clinical description. Ann Surg 117: 834–864
2. Benzer H, Haider W, Mutz N, Geyer A, Goldschmied W, Pauser G, Baum M (1979) Der alveolo-arterielle Sauerstoffquotient = „Quotient" = PAO_2-PaO_2/PAO_2. Anaesthesist 28: 533–539
3. Bone RC, Fisher CJ, Clemmer TP, Slotman GJ, Metz CA, Balk RA (1990) Sepsis syndrom: a valid clinical entity. Crit Care Med 17: 389–393
4. Bull JP, Squire JR (1949) A study of mortality in a burn unit: standards for the evaluation of alternative methods of treatment. Ann Surg 130: 160
5. Clark CJ, Reid WH, Telfer ABM, Campbell D (1983) Respiratory injury in the burned patient. The role of flexible bronchoscopy. Anaesthesia 38: 35–39
6. Clark WR Jr, Nieman GF (1988) Smoke inhalation. Burns 14: 473–494
7. Davies LK, Poulton TJ, Modell JH (1983) Continuous positive airway pressure is beneficial in treatment of smoke inhalation. Crit Care Med 11: 726–729
8. Epstein BS, Hardy D, Harrison HN, Teplitz C, Villarreal Y, Mason AD (1963) Hypoxemia in the burned patient: a clinical-pathologic study. Ann Surg 158: 924–932
9. Fein A, Leff A, Hopewell PC (1980) Pathophysiology and management of the complications resulting from fire and the inhaled products of combustion. Crit Care Med 8: 94–98
10. Feller I, Flora JD, Bawol R (1976) Baseline results of therapy for burned patients. JAMA 236: 1943–1947
11. Gillespie DJ, Marsh HMM, Divertie MB, Meadows JA (1986) Clinical outcome of respiratory failure in patients requiring prolonged (>24 hours) mechanical ventilation. Chest 90: 364–369
12. Hunt JL, Agee RN, Pruitt BA Jr (1975) Fiberoptic bronchoscopy in acute inhalation injury. J Trauma 15: 641–648
13. Kaukinen L, Pasanen M, Kaukinen S (1985) Prognostic indicators in burned patients. Ann Chirurg Gynaecol 74: 86–89
14. Luce EA, Su CT, Hoopes JE (1976) Alveolar-arterial oxygen gradient in the burn patient. J Trauma 16: 212–217
15. Mallory TB, Brickley WJ (1943) Pathology: with special reference to the pulmonary lesions. Ann Surg 117: 865–884
16. McManus WF, Goodwin CW, Mason AD Jr, Pruitt BA Jr (1981) Burn wound infection. J Trauma 21: 753–756
17. Meck M, Munster AM, Winchurch RA, Dickerson C (1991) The Baltimore sepsis scale: measurement of sepsis on patients with burns using a new scoring system. J Burn Care Rehabil 12: 564–568

18. Moylan JA, Alexander LG Jr (1978) Diagnosis and treatment of inhalation injury. World J Surg 2:185–191
19. Peterson VM, Murphy JR, Haddix T, Ford P, Anderson JA, Bartle EJ (1988) Identification of novel prognostic indicators in burned patients. J Trauma 28:632–637
20. Phillips AW, Cope O (1962) The relevation of respiratory tract damage as a principal killer of the burned patient. Ann Surg 155:1–19
21. Prien T, Traber DL (1988) Toxic smoke compounds and inhalation injury – a review. Burns 14:451–460
22. Scott-Conner CEH, Coil JA, Conner HF, Mack ME (1986) Wound closure index: A guide to prognosis in burned patients. J Trauma 26:123–127
23. Scott-Conner CEH, Meydrech E, Wheeler WE, Coil JA (1988) Quantitation of rate of wound closure and the prediction of death following major burns. Burns 14:373–378
24. Shirani KZ, Pruitt BA, Mason AD (1987) The influence of inhalation injury and pneumonia on burn mortality. Ann Surg 205:82–87
25. Stern M, Waisbren BA (1979) Comparison of methods of predicting burn mortality. Burns 6:119–123
26. Stuttmann R, Knüttgen D, Eichler F, Doehn M (1985) Das Inhalationstrauma. Differentialdiagnose und Prognose. Anaesthesist [Suppl] 34:265
27. Stuttmann R, Knüttgen D, Müller MR, Spilker G, Doehn M (1989) Die prognostische Bedeutung der Gasaustauschstörung beim Inhalationstrauma. Anaesthesist [Suppl] 38:696
28. Tejerina C, Reig A, Codina J, Safont J, Mirabet V (1992) Burns in patients over 60 years old: epidemiology and mortality. Burns 18:149–152
29. Thompson PB, Herndon DN, Traber DL, Abston S (1986) Effect on mortality of inhalation injury. J Trauma 26:136–165
30. Tobiasen J, Hiebert JH, Edlich RF (1982) A practical burn severity index. J Burn Care Rehab 3:229–232
31. Tobiasen J, Hiebert JH, Edlich RF (1982) Prediction of burn mortality. Surg Gynecol Obstet 154:711–714
32. Traber DL, Linares HA, Herndon DN, Prien T (1988) The pathophysiology of inhalation injury – a review. Burns 14:357–364
33. Tredget EE, Shankowsky HA, Taerum TV, Moysa GL, Alton JDM (1990) The role of inhalation injury in burn trauma. Ann Surg 212:720–727
34. Zawacki BE, Azen SP, Imbus SH, Chang YC (1979) Multifactorial probit analysis of mortality in burned patients. Ann Surg 189:1–5

Anschrift des Verfassers:
Dr. R. Stuttmann
Kliniken der Stadt Köln
Krankenhaus Merheim
Ostmerheimer Straße 200
D-51109 Köln 91

Microbial translocation following burn injury

J. W. Alexander and L. Gianotti

Department of Surgery, University of Cincinnati College of Medicine, Cincinnati, Ohio, USA

Microbial translocation is defined as the passage of both viable and nonviable microbes and microbial products across the intact intestinal barrier [1]. Most of the time, translocation has been measured by simply culturing microorganisms from different tissues or fluids. Using this technique, the amount of viable organisms in the tissues that results in translocation is determined by three factors: 1) the number and types of microbes in the intestinal lumen, i.e., the greater the number of bacteria in the lumen the greater will be the degree of translocation; 2) the rate of passage across the mucosal barrier (the translocation process itself), and 3) the clearance of the bacteria by host defense mechanisms from the tissues.

In studying the translocation process, several facts should be kept in mind. One is that human feces and feces of other mammals contain a large number of bacterial species which reach very high concentrations in the stool, as many as 10^{12} organisms per gram of stool. In humans, the anaerobes outnumber aerobes about 100:1 and even more in several animal species. The small bowel absorptive surface in an adult man is about 2 million cm^2 which is more than 100 times the skin surface area and equal to the size of a single tennis court. One can then imagine a quantity of bacteria, equal to more than 1000 times the number of humans on the earth, trying to escape from the intestinal lumen to the other side of the gut wall.

The mechanisms of microbial translocation

Studies were done in burned guinea pigs with an exteriorized Thiry-Vella loop into which *Candida albicans* were placed immediately before the time of a burn injury [1]. The animals were sacrificed at different intervals thereafter and scanning electron micrographs made of the loop. The results showed that clumps of *Candida albicans* initially become attached irregularly to villi soon after the burn injury, probably by a biochemical mechanism involving receptors, although this has not been extensively explored at the present time. By transmission electron microscopy (TEM), it was possible to observe a dissolution of the microvilli as candida organisms became attached. Shortly after attachment, disorganization at the tips of the microvilli was noticed as if there was an enzymatic process which could cause this type of penetration into the layer (Fig. 1). In many histologic samples groups of *Candida albicans* could be seen partly penetrating into the microvillus layer. In some of the scanning electron microscopy specimens it was possible to see circular defects of the brush border. These kinds of superficial lesions of the microvillus layer were very probably caused by attached candida stripped off during the process of tissue preparation

---

Supported by USPHS Grant No. AI12936

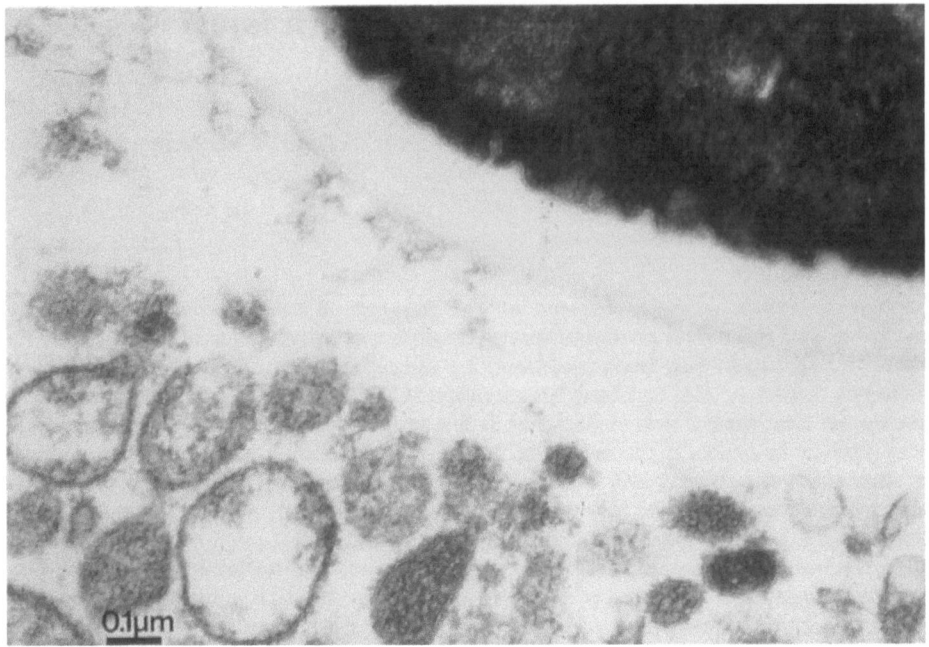

Fig. 1. Attachment of *Candida albicans* to the microvillus layer of the ileum shows some disruption of the microvilli at the point of contact

(Fig. 2). On other samples, single candidal bodies were seen attached to the microvillus layer while other Candida were already penetrating.

By TEM, it was possible to observe the disturbance of the microvilli more closely and appreciate that they become disorganized and sometimes shrunken (Fig. 3). Often, fragments of microvilli became attached to the outer surface of candidal bodies as they moved through the brush border layer toward the outer membrane of the cells. Sometimes, the process of penetration was associated with a hyperplastic response of the microvilli. The dynamic process of translocation was demonstrable in many samples that showed numerous candida in the microvillus layer as well as within enterocytes. By TEM, we were able to localize the point at which candidal organisms had entered the plasma membrane, but we have not seen one actually passing through the membrane, indicating that this is a very rapid process. Apparently, the membrane opens up and lets the organism in without the development of a phagocytic membrane. There is no membrane surrounding the organisms when they are in the enterocyte. However, the candida may drag in remnants of microvilli from the outside. At higher magnifications, we never observed direct evidence of cytoplasmic injury to the cell, evidence of degranulation within the cell, or evidence of any interaction with the intracellular structures and bodies within the candidal organism.

In one extraordinary example, candida were seen passing from the apical to the basal portion of a particular enterocyte at the same time that two macrophages were exiting the mucosa through the intercellular junctions. The passage of the organisms

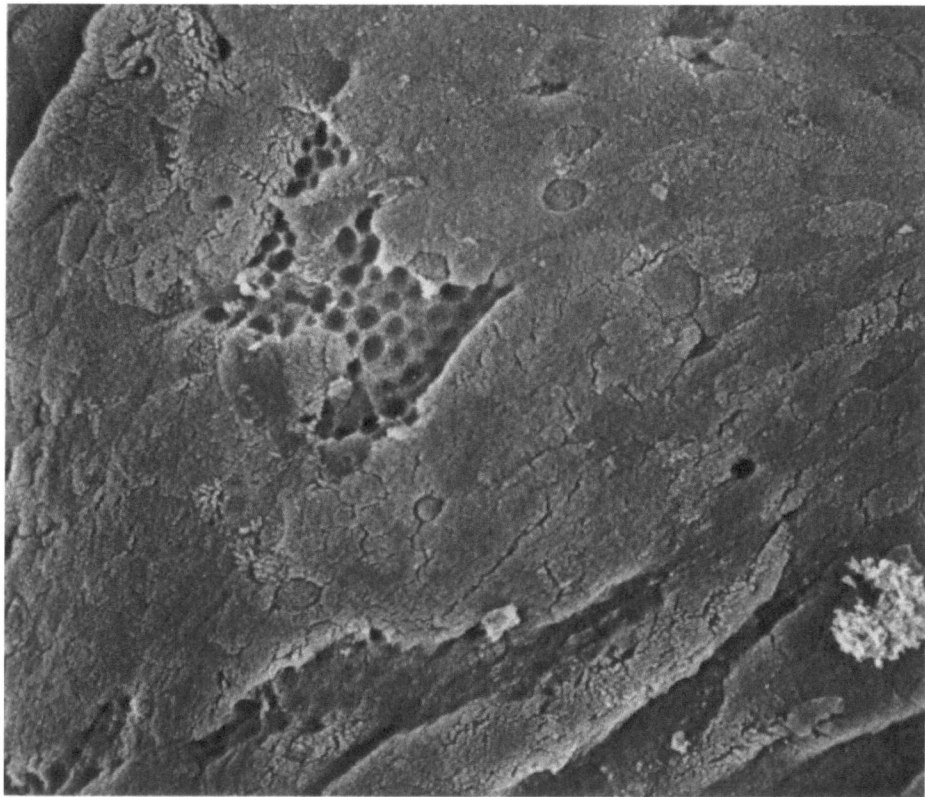

Fig. 2. Scanning electron micrograph of the mucosal layer of a burned animal with candida introduced into a Thiry-Vella loop shows a group of eroded areas where candida have partially penetrated into the microvillus layer. The candida had been dislodged during preparation of the sample

by translocation into the lamina propria is always through the cytoplasm and never between the enterocytes, although the exit of macrophages occurs between the cells. Finally, when the candida reached the basal surface of the enterocytes, the basal membrane simply opened up and the organisms were extruded into the lamina propria by a process different from exocytosis since *C. albicans* did not have a containing membrane around them [1]. Very similar observations were done in the human small intestine. Candida organisms were placed into the lumen of the intestine of a cadaver donor before placing the gut on normothermic perfusion. *Candida albicans* were seen translocating through the intact mucosa and entering the lamina propria. After entry into the lamina propria, the organisms may be carried into the lymphatics or venules free or within macrophages and pass to different parts of the body.

Translocation of *E. coli* occurs by exactly the same mechanism described for *C. albicans*, passing through and not between the epithelial cells [1, 2]. Subsequently, the organisms get into the lamina propria and are taken up by macrophages. Free endotoxin, as well as *E. coli* may pass through the muscular layer of the intestine wall

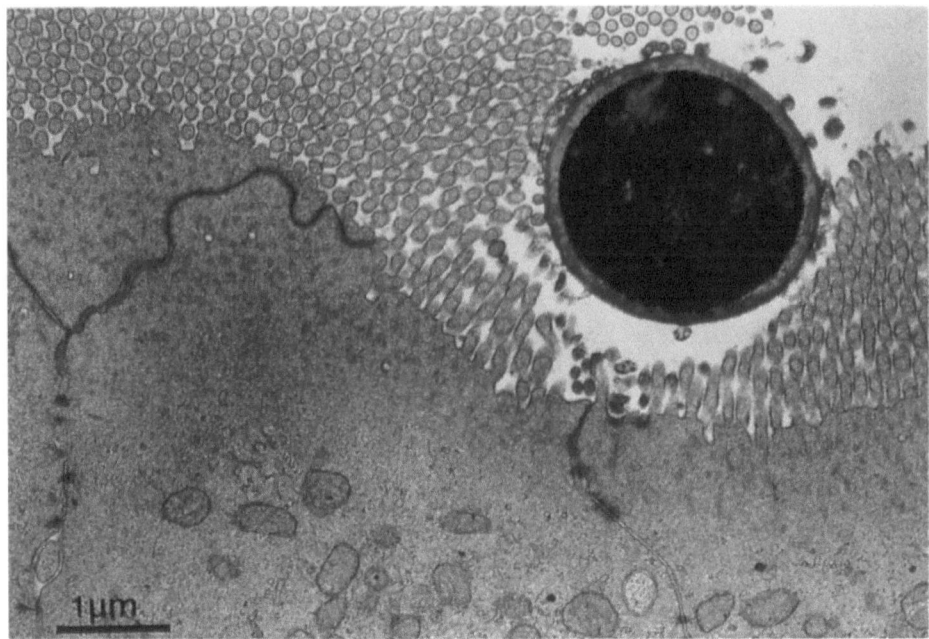

Fig. 3. Transmission electron microscopy of a candidal body almost completely embedded in the microvillus layer. Disorganization of the microvilli adjacent to the candida is evident with fragments of the microvilli becoming attached to the outer portion of the candidal body

between the myocytes rather than through them. By this mechanism, the peritoneal cavity may be contaminated with viable organisms in absence of defects in the mucosal structure.

The process of translocation, studied extensively by Deitch and his colleagues [3, 4], has been shown by Herndon et al. [6, 9] to be related to blood flow to the intestine. In a particularly interesting experiment, we were able to show that, by counting the number of translocating candida within an individual villus and the number of microspheres trapped in each villus after injection into the arterial circulation, there was an inverse correlation between the two parameters. As the number of microspheres increased, indicating an increased blood flow to the individual villus, the number of candida translocating to that villus decreased. These findings suggested a very strong relationship between the microcirculation to each individual villus, as well as the gross splanchnic circulation to the intestine.

Patterns of Distribution and Clearance of Translocating Organisms after Burn Injury

In one set of experiments, *E. coli* was labeled with ^{14}C glucose placed in a glucose free culture medium so that the organism could be labeled intrinsically [2]. Mice were then gavaged with 1×10^8 labeled *E. coli*, and a 30% total body surface area burn injury was inflicted. The animals were sacrificed at 1, 4, and 24 h after the time of burn injury and different tissues were harvested to measure residual radioactivity. As might be expected, the mesenteric lymph nodes had the highest concentration of translocation. Within 1 h of burn injury there was extensive translocation to the mesenteric lymph nodes as well as other tissue. Radioactivity in the tissue persisted over 24 h even though there was a dynamic process that allowed bacteria to leave the lymph nodes and bring in more translocated material. The spleen and lung also had a relatively high level of translocation and there was even significant translocation to the peritoneal cavity through the intact muscular wall. By measuring the percentage of organisms that remained viable in the tissues (as calculated by the difference between cultured organisms and radioactivity), a very rapid clearance of the bacteria could be appreciated. The most rapid killing was in the mesenteric lymph nodes, spleen, blood, and peritoneal cavity with less rapid clearance in the liver and lung. Using 100 times more organisms for gavage (10^{10}), a similar pattern was seen with minor differences. There was very rapid entrance into the mesenteric lymph nodes and spleen, with a little less in the liver, lung, and blood, and persistence over 24 h. Using this higher dose, the clearance, as measured by the percent of viable organisms remaining was less in the lung and in the peritoneal cavity, but was very rapid in the mesenteric lymph nodes; less than one in 1000 organisms remained viable in the mesenteric lymph nodes and spleen.

Using ^{14}C endotoxin which we extracted from ^{14}C radioisotope labeled organisms, it was possible to see a similar pattern of translocation. There was rapid entrance of the labeled endotoxin to the mesenteric lymph nodes, but somewhat less to the spleen and more to the liver and lung. However, in these experiments, the lung data must be analyzed with caution because there could have been some spillover into the lung at the time of gavage.

Effects of Burn Size

Another set of experiments using ^{14}C radiolabeled *E. coli* was done to determine the distribution, not only to the organs, but also to the burn eschar following thermal injury of different body surface areas [5]. Minimal translocation was seen to the liver and mesenteric lymph nodes in both normal and awake animals, and in animals receiving anesthesia. Animals with a 10% burn, 20% burn, and 30% burn showed increasing translocation to all of the tissues, but a 50% burn was associated with a lesser degree of translocation than a 30% burn. This is consistent with the hypothesis that the translocation process is energy dependent and that injury can be sufficiently severe to limit the availability of energy for transport of organisms across the intestinal epithelium. In contrast, the clearance of live *E. coli* translocated to the various tissues was progressively inhibited with increasing size of burn injury, suggesting that the host's ability to kill translocating bacteria is inversely related to the severity of trauma. The data also show that enteric organisms can populate the burn eschar by the blood stream.

Effects of Nutrition

Additional studies were undertaken to determine whether nutrient intake early after injury would alter gut barrier function to bacteria. In one experiment, Balb/c mice (nine per group) were deprived of food for 0, 6, 12, 18, or 24 h before gavage with

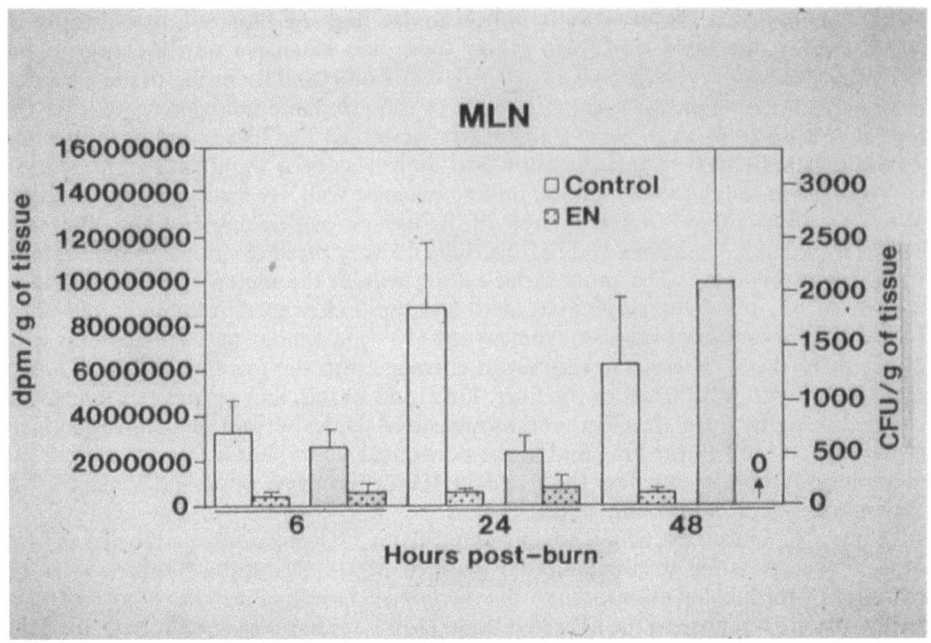

Fig. 4. Concentrations of radionuclide and viable organisms in mesenteric lymph nodes of animals with a 50% burn injury 6, 24, or 48 h after the onset of enteral nutrition or Ringer's lactate infusion. EN – animals fed immediately after injury (stipped bars). See text for details

1×10^{14} ^{14}C labeled *E. coli*. Immediately thereafter, a 30% burn injury was inflicted under general anesthesia and the animals were sacrificed 4 h later. As measured by the radioactivity reaching the mesenteric lymph nodes, there was a progressive increase in translocation with starvation. In contrast, however, the number of colony-forming units per gram of tissue and the percentage of bacteria which remained alive decreased with food deprivation, indicating that although there was an impairment of the epithelial barrier, the host defense mechanisms were progressively more able to clear translocated bacteria. Similar findings were observed in the spleen, liver, and other tissues. In another experiment, guinea pigs had gastrostomies placed surgically and they were allowed to recover for 7–10 days during which time they regained their preoperative weight. Under general anesthesia, a 40% burn was then inflicted and animals were randomly assigned to two groups. In the first group, a complete liquid enteral diet was instituted immediately after burn injury and in the second group, Ringer's lactate solution in the same volume was started immediately after injury via gastrostomy. Subgroups of eight animals were then given 1×10^{10} ^{14}C labeled *E. coli* by gastrostomy 6, 24, or 48 h after the onset of enteral nutrition

---

Fig. 5. a Relationship between plasma glucagon and jejunal mucosal weight 24 h after burn injury. Some animals had received early enteral feeding whereas others had not. Note the strong inverse relationship between mucosal weight and plasma glucagon levels for individual animals. Adapted from [8] with permission. **b** Relationship between plasma cortisol and jejunal mucosal weight 24 h after burn injury. The same relationships are noted. Adapted from [8], with permission

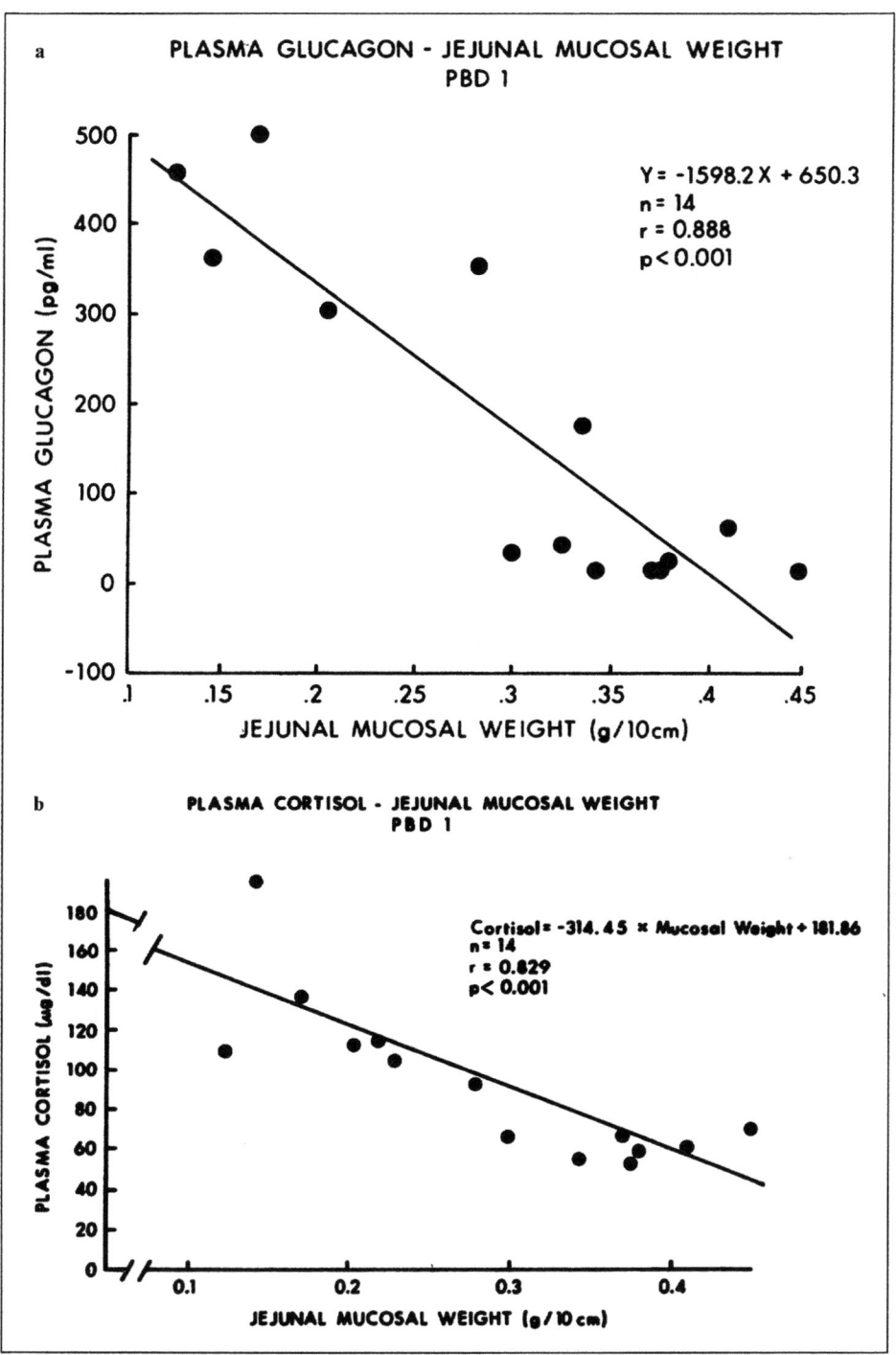

or Ringer's lactate infusion, and they were sacrificed 4 h afterwards. Six hours after injury, the animals given Ringer's lactate solution had approximately 80%–90% more translocation to the mesenteric lymph nodes and other tissues than did fed animals (Fig. 4). Translocation in nonfed animals increased another three-fold by 24 h and stayed high, whereas the amount of translocation in fed animals, as measured by radionuclide counts in the mesenteric lymph nodes, remained basically stable. Colony-forming units of *E. coli.*, however, were found to be progressively higher at 48 h in nonfed animals, while no viable bacteria were culturable in the animals that were fed immediately after burn injury. Analysis of radionuclide counts and colony forming units in the lung and other tissues followed a similar pattern. It could be concluded from these experiments that food deprivation without injury for up to 24 hrs significantly increased the rate of translocation to mesenteric lymph nodes and only modestly to the spleen or liver. However, in all tissues there was increased killing of translocated bacteria. Thus, thermal injury markedly increased the rate of microbial translocation across the mucosal barrier, but early enteral nutrition strikingly decreased the rate of translocation at 6, 24, and 48 h after burn injury. Food deprivation after injury resulted in decreased clearance of translocating bacteria from the tissue as early as 24 h postburn by improving host defense mechanisms.

Previous studies have shown that early enteral feeding may decrease the hypermetabolic response to injury and the secretion of catabolic hormones. We reported in 1984 that early enteral feeding decreased the hypermetabolic rate by approximately 80% in guinea pigs with a 30% burn compared to animals which had restricted enteral feeding during the first 3 days [8]. In animals given only lactated Ringer's during the first 24 h, plasma cortisol levels more than doubled. In contrast, this increase was only approximately 10% above normal controls in animals given early enteral feedings. The mucosal weight of the jejunum decreased by almost 50% during the first 24 h after burn injury in animals given only lactated Ringer's solution by the enteral route. Conversely, the mucosal weight did not decrease significantly in animals fed immediately after burn injury. Both plasma cortisol and glucagon increased dramatically after burn injury without enteral feeding and both plasma cortisol and plasma glucagon levels had striking inverse relationships with jejunal mucosal weight when individual animals were plotted on a scattergram (Fig. 5).

The above studies also strongly suggest that early feedings will decrease the incidence of infection. This hypothesis is, perhaps, best endorsed by a study of Kudsk et al. [7]. Patients with severe trauma who had laparotomies were provided with both feeding jejunostomies and central venous lines at the time of the operative procedure. They were then randomly assigned to receive either early enteral feedings or total parenteral nutrition. Forty-one percent of the patients receiving TPN developed an infectious episode compared to 15% of the patients receiving enteral nutrition ($p<0.03$), and 49% of patients receiving TPN developed pneumonia compared to 6% receiving enteral nutrition ($p<0.01$).

Conclusion

Microbial translocation from the intestine following burn injury is an important cause of infectious complications and can lead to both a hypermetabolic state and clinical sepsis. Early enteral feeding with a complete enteral diet after burn injury can reduce translocation, infectious complications, hypermetabolic responses, and hospital stay.

References

1. Alexander JW, Boyce ST, Babcock GF, Gianotti L, Peck M, Dunn DL, Pyles T, Childress CP, Ash SK (1990) The process of microbial translocation. Ann Surg 212:496–512
2. Alexander JW, Gianotti L, Pyles T, Carey MA, Babcock GF (1991) Distribution and survival of *Escherichia coli* translocating from the intestine after thermal injury. Ann Surg 213:558–566
3. Deitch EA, Berg R (1987) Bacterial translocation from the gut: a mechanism of infection. J Burn Care Rehab 8:475–483
4. Deitch EA, Ma WJ, Ma L, Berg R, Specian RD (1989) Endotoxin-induced bacterial translocation: a study of mechanisms. Surgery 106:292–300
5. Gianotti L, Pyles T, Alexander JW, James L, Babcock GF. Relationship between extent of burn injury and magnitude of microbial translocation from the intestine. J Burn Care Rehab, in press
6. Herndon DN, Morris SE, Coffey JA (1989) Enteric translocation of microorganisms in cutaneous thermal injury. Proc Clin Biol Res 308:377–382
7. Kudsk KA, Croce MA, Fabian TC, Minard G, Tolley EA, Poret III A, Kuhl MR, Brown RD (1992) Enteral versus parenteral feeding: effects on septic morbidity following blunt and penetrating abdominal trauma. Ann Surg 215 (5):503–513
8. Mochizuki H, Trocki O, Dominioni L, Brackett KA, Joffe SN, Alexander JW (1984) Mechanism of prevention of postburn hypermetabolism and catabolism by early enteral feeding. Ann Surg 200:297–308
9. Morris SE, Navaratnam N, Herndon DN (1990) A comparison of effect of thermal injury and smoke inhalation on bacterial translocation. J Trauma 30:639–645

Authors' address:
J. Wesley Alexander, M.D.
Department of Surgery
University of Cincinnati College of Medicine
231 Bethesda Avenue, Cincinnati
Ohio 45267-0558 U.S.A.

Therapie

Topical and surgical treatment of the burn wound

D. N. Herndon, R. L. Rutan and T. C. Rutan

Shriners Burns Institute, Galveston, Texas, USA

Regardless of the source of burn injury, the end result is coagulation of tissue, initiation of an inflammatory cascade, and a systemic "reset" of metabolic and immunologic profiles. Any concomitant injury superimposes additional changes to those already instigated by the burn wound itself.

Treatment of the burn wound has traditionally revolved around topical therapies. Throughout the ages, various substances have been applied to the burn wound to encourage healing. Some of these "folk remedies" continue to be used in various parts of the world and some have been demonstrated to be of benefit (Aloe, tannic acid). However, it was not until the introduction of topical antimicrobial agents that a significant decrease in the mortality related to burn injuries was realized.

Colonization (bacterial or fungal) of the burn wound eschar and granulating surfaces present a constant potential reservoir of microbes and their byproducts. There is a consensus that attempts to make and maintain the wound sterile are unrealistic as contamination may occur from both exogenous and endogenous sources. However, it is realistic to control the microbiologic flora with the prophylactic use of topical agents.

Topical antimicrobial agents are used from the time of admission, and include mafenide acetate [24], silver sulfadiazine [10], gentamicin [23], 0.5% silver nitrate [25], povidone iodine [27], nitrofurazone [11], and nystatin [30]. The effectiveness of any of these agents is related to their ability to inhibit bacterial growth in vitro and reduce colony counts in vivo. Studies have documented the ineffectiveness of silver nitrate, nitrofurazone and povidone iodine to inhibit bacterial growth in agar diffusion studies [18]. No single agent is totally effective against all burn wound microorganisms, therefore treatment should be guided by in vitro testing or in vivo results. We perform quantitative and qualitative eschar and granulating wound biopsies three times weekly, obtaining one sample for every 18% body surface area open. Gram stain and rapid histologic biopsy are obtained at times when there is clinical suspicion of burn wound sepsis, if the contaminating wound has not been cultured recently.

Our topical agent of choice is silver sulfadiazine. Deep partial thickness wounds are treated with this substance until healing, or until colony counts exceed 10^3 organisms/g tissue. When colony counts rise to that level, we empirically change to mafenide acetate, due to its broad spectrum effect and its ability to diffuse through the wound to the systemic circulation [12, 13]. Full thickness wounds are treated with silver sulfadiazine preoperatively, as we treat full thickness injuries with early excision and grafting.

The use of any topical antimicrobial agent inhibits the rate of wound re-epithelialization. Biologic dressings such as porcine xenograft (pigskin) and cadaveric allograft (homograft), have been noted to adhere to the wound surface [4], reduce wound colony counts [5], decrease transcutaneous fluid and protein losses [21] and reduce pain.

Pigskin serves as well as cadaver skin in all functions except when used following burn wound excision. Pigskin, as currently available in the US, is not living and will not vascularize [29]. Indications for the use of biologic dressings are: 1) immediate coverage of superficial fully debrided partial thickness burn wounds, 2) coverage of granulating excised wounds while autograft donor sites are healing, 3) as a test graft before autograft application, and 4) debridement of granulating wounds with adherent necrotic tissue [26].

Application of pigskin to fresh partial thickness wounds provides a physiologic environment for re-epithelialization. Partial thickness wounds treated with biologic dressings, Biobrane or OpSite heal at a faster rate than wounds treated with mafenide acetate or silver sulfadiazine [6]. Both homograft and xenograft, when allowed to adhere to the wound, promote epithelial cell proliferation. As keratinization of the healed epithelium occurs, the biologic dressing is sloughed. The success of this process is dependent upon the adherence of the biologic dressing to the wound and the cleanliness of the wound itself. Any necrotic tissue remaining under the dressing will create a closed fluid loculation, which can become infected and destroy the remaining epithelial structures, converting a partial thickness wound to a full thickness one. We routinely use cadaveric allograft on partial thickness scald injuries [9].

Early surgical removal of full thickness eschar falls into one of the basic tenets of surgery, "Separate the patient from the disease". Historically, the burn wound has been allowed to remain in situ and to spontaneously separate from the viable granulating bed [2]. More recently, controlled excision of small portions of the burn wound have been performed in a staged manner [19, 7].

We combine the technique of early tangential excision introduced by Janzekovic [20] and those of Burke [3] and Alexander [1] for wound closure. Since excision of large amounts of surface area will not allow for complete autologous closure, we frequently use cadaveric allograft as a temporary wound closure. Alternately, allograft is used to physiologically close widely meshed autograft [15]. Using this technique, we have demonstrated improved survival statistics in children when massive excision was performed early in the postburn period [14]. However, the salutary effects noted in the pediatric patient have failed to translate to the adult population.

Early excision is performed at the expense of some viable tissue. The amount of viable tissue loss is dependent upon the depth of excision. Obvious, deep, subdermal injuries are carried out to the level of fascia and obvious partial thickness injuries may be adequately debrided with tangential escharectomy. The removal of large surface area injuries must be conducted with consideration of blood loss, the patient's preoperative condition, and the depth of injury. The possibility of improved cosmetics in deep tangential vs. excision to fat vs. fascial excision must also be considered. In general, we reserve fascial excision for the deep, massive injuries, in full knowledge that some viable tissue may be sacrificed in the attempt to save the patient.

There is a temporal relationship between blood loss and the timing of excision. In a study of 594 patients, we demonstrated a 50% decrease in blood loss if excision was performed within the first 24 h postburn as opposed to excising after 24 h postburn, but before 16 days postburn [8]. The results of this study make a strong argument for this procedure, especially in the face of massive burns where significant blood loss is unavoidable.

Such an aggressive approach must be undertaken with full awareness of the hemodynamic and pathophysiologic changes ongoing in the acute resuscitation period. Intensive and expert monitoring of intravascular volume status is essential. Urine output should be monitored via an indwelling Foley catheter and an intraoperative urine output of 0.75 ml/kg/h is considered indicative of adequate renal perfusion and is a useful guide to judge the overall fluid status. Blood loss should be replaced ml/ml with whole blood equivalent. The only crystalloid administered to the patient should be their calculated resuscitation requirements.

Ideally, all excised wounds would be covered with autograft sheets or mesh of minimal expansion. This would maximize both cosmetic and functional results while minimizing the exposure to burn wound sepsis by closing the wound. Unfortunately, this goal is rarely achieved in all but minor injuries. This necessitates the utilization of compromise measures including grafts meshed and expanded to a 1:1.5, 1:2, 1:3 or even 1:4 ratio. Some authors [22] have advocated extremely thin 1:6 and 1:9 expansions in emergency circumstances as life-saving procedures. The value of such widely expanded skin is debatable as the resultant epidermis is very thin and highly susceptible to sheering forces and minimal trauma. Sheet grafts should be employed, whenever possible, in areas of vital function (e.g., the hands) and prominent cosmetics (e.g., face, ears, neck).

Wounds grafted with $>1:2$ expanded skin or excised wounds for which autograft is not available are best covered with a biologic dressing. We prefer fresh frozen cadaver skin; however, synthetic covers and xenograft have been used. Widely expanded autograft ($\geq 1:4$) is best closed physiologically with 1:2 expanded allograft overlay as this provides a barrier to bacterial invasion, decreases evaporative water loss and prevents wound desiccation while offering minimal resistance to epithelialization [24, 6]. The allograft overlay adheres to the open interstices, allowing vascularization and endogenous bacterial killing. When insufficient autograft is available, allograft may be used to close the remaining excised wounds. In patients with large burn injuries, donor sites can be successfully recropped every 5–7 days, until all cadaver skin is replaced. Even burns of $>98\%$ TBSA can be closed with this technique.

We have had favorable results using this aggressive technique. Blood loss, length of hospital stay, and mortality (in children and young adults) have decreased. With physiologic closure of the excised wound, there is a decrease or stabilization of fluid losses, subjective pain, and wound infections. We thought that closure of the metabolically active burn wound would reduce or eliminate the hypermetabolic response. Unfortunately, early closure of the burn wound, in our experience, has not abolished the postburn hypermetabolic response.

A prospective, randomized study of 13 burn patients with $>40\%$ TBSA revealed no significant differences in energy expenditure, respiratory quotient or oxygen consumption between those treated by early excision and those treated conservatively [28]. Our attempts to moderate the hypermetabolic response using propranolol [16], which decreased heart rate but maintained cardiac output, and recombinant human growth hormone [17], which allowed more rapid closure of the burn wound, have been unsuccessful; metabolic rate remained unchanged.

In sum, control of wound flora can be achieved with the use of prophylactic topical antimicrobial agents. Aggressive surveillance measures are required to maintain microbial control. Use of topical agents must be guided by in vitro testing and in vivo results. Biologic dressings provide a physiologic environment for epithelial cell proliferation. As the epithelium proliferates the adherent biologic dressing is sloughed; however, the success of the process depends upon the cleanliness of the wound and the adherence of the dressing. Early surgical excision allows the patient to be separated from the disease. Large excisional and grafting procedures can be routinely and safely performed within the first 24 h postburn and save 50% of the blood loss when compared to excisions done between 1–16 days postburn. Early excision decreases length of hospital stay and improves mortality, but has had no effect in eliminating the hypermetabolic response to trauma.

References

1. Alexander JW, MacMillan BG, Law E (1981) Treatment of severe burns with widely meshed skin autograft and meshed skin allograft overlay. J Trauma 21:433
2. Blocker TG (1954) Late treatment of severe extensive burns. South Med J 47:371
3. Burke JF, Conrado BC, Quimby WC (1974) Primary burn excision and immediate grafting: a method of shortening illness. J Trauma 14:389
4. Burleson R, Eisemann B (1972) Nature of the bond between partial thickness skin and wound granulations. Surg 72(2):315
5. Burleson R, Eisemann B (1973) Mechanisms of antibacterial effect of biologic dressings. Ann Surg 177–181
6. Burleson R, Eisemann E (1973) Effect of skin dressings and topical antimicrobics on healing of partial thickness skin wounds in rats. Surg Gynecol Obstet 136:158
7. Cramer LM; McCormack RM, Carroll DB (1962) Progressive partial excision and early grafting in lethal burns. Plast Reconstr Surg 30:595
8. Desai MH, Herndon DN, Broemeling LD et al. (1990) Early burn wound excision significantly reduces blood loss. Ann Surg 211(6):753
9. Desai MH, Rutan RL, Herndon DN (1991) Conservative treatment of scald burns is superior to early excision. J Burn Bare & Rehabil 12(5): 482
10. Fox JCL, Rappole BW, Stanford W (1969) Control of pseudomonas infection in burns by silver sulfadiazine. Surg Gynecol Obstet 12S:1021
11. Georgiade N, Lucas M, Georgiade R, et al. (1967) The use of new potent topical antibacterial agent for the control of infection in the burn wound. Plast Reconstr. Surg 39:349
12. Harrison HN, Bales H, Jacoby F (1971) The behavior of mafenide acetate as a basis for its clinical use. Arch Surg 103:449
13. Harrison HN; Blackmore WP, Bales HW, et al. (1972) The absorption of C-14 labeled sulfamylon acetate through burned skin: 1. Experimental methods and initial observations. J Trauma 12:986
14. Herndon DN, Parks DH (1986) Comparison of serial debridement and autografting and early massive excision with cadaver skin overlay in the treatment of large burns in children. J Trauma 26:149
15. Herndon DN, Barrow RE, Rutan RL et al (1989) A comparison of conservative versus early excision. Ann Surg 209(5):547
16. Herndon DN, Barrow RE, Rutan TC, Minifee P, Johoor F, Wolfe RR (1988) Effect of propranolol administration on hemodynamic and metabolic responses of burned pediatric patients. Ann Surg 208(4):484–492
17. Herndon DN, Barrow RE, Kunkel KR, Broemeling LD, Rutan RL (1990) Effect of recombinant human growth hormone on donor site healing in severely burned children. Ann Surg 212(4):424–431
18. Holder IA, Schwab M; Jackson L (1979) Eighteen months of routine topical antimicrobial susceptibility testing of isolates from burn patients: Results and conclusions. J Antibicrob Chemother 5:455

19. Jackson D (1953) The diagnosis of depth of burning. Br J Surg 40:588
20. Janzekovic Z (1970) A new concept in early excision and immediate grafting of burns. J Trauma 10:1102
21. Lamke LO, Nilsson GE, Reithner HS (1978) The evaporative water loss from burns and the water vapor permeability of grafts and artificial membranes used in the treatment of burns. Burns 3:159
22. MacMillan BG (1967) Early excision. J Trauma 7:75–79
23. MacMillan BG (1971) Ecology of bacteria colonizing the burned patient given topical and systemic gentamicin therapy: a five year study. J Infect Dis 124:5278
24. Moncrief JA, Lindberg RB, Switzer WE et al (1966) Use of topical antibacterial therapy in the treatment of the burn wound. Arch Surg 92:558
25. Moyer CA, Brentano L, Gravens DL et al (1956) Treatment of large human burns with 0.5% silver nitrate solution. Arch Surg 90:812
26. Pruitt BA Jr, Curreri PW (1971) The use of homograft and heterograft skin. In: Polk HC, Stone H (Eds). *Contemporary Burn Management*. Boston, Little Brown and Co.
27. Robson MC, Schaerf RHM, Krizek TJ (1974) Evaluation of topical povidone iodine ointment in experimental burn wound sepsis. Plast Reconstr Surg 54:328
28. Rutan TC, Herndon DN, VanOsten T, Abston S (1986) Metabolic rate alterations in early excision and grafting versus conservative treatment. J Trauma 26(2):140–142
29. Shuck JM (1977) The use of heteroplastic grafts. Burns 2:47
30. Stone HH, Kolb LD, Currie CA et al. (1974) Candida sepsis: Pathogenesis and principles of treatment. Ann Surg 179(5):697

Author's address:
David N. Herndon, MD
Shriners Burns Institute
815 Market St
Galveston, TX 77550, USA

Die konservative und operative Therapie der Brandwunde

P. R. Zellner, T. Raff und S. Lorenz

BG Unfallklinik Ludwigshafen, Abt. für Verbrennungen,
plastische und Handchirurgie (Chefarzt: Prof. Dr. Dr. P. R. Zellner)

Krankheitsverlauf und Prognose schwerer Verbrennungen werden in entscheidendem Maße davon bestimmt, ob es gelingt, das Auftreten septischer Komplikationen zu verhindern. Als Ursache solcher Komplikationen spielt neben der Pneumonie, den Katheterinfektionen und der Invasion von pathogenen Keimen aus dem Darm die Wundinfektion eine hervorragende Rolle (Abb. 1). Deshalb ist die Behandlung der Brandwunde zusammen mit Maßnahmen der Asepsis und Antisepsis zentrales Problem der Verbrennungstherapie (Abb. 2).

Schon im vergangenen Jahrhundert kannte man eine große Anzahl unterschiedlicher Oberflächenbehandlungsmittel, die eine Infektion verhindern und den Wundverschluß fördern sollten. Die zum Teil schwersten Nebenwirkungen einiger Substanzen, insbesondere des Tannins, brachten die topische Wundbehandlung vorübergehend in Verruf, und erst in den 60er Jahren wurden Oberflächenbehandlungsmittel wieder systematisch angewandt. Besonders erfolgreich waren das Sulfamylon, das Silber-Sulfadiazin, die Gropp'sche Gerbung und das PVP-Jod. Die an ein Oberflä-

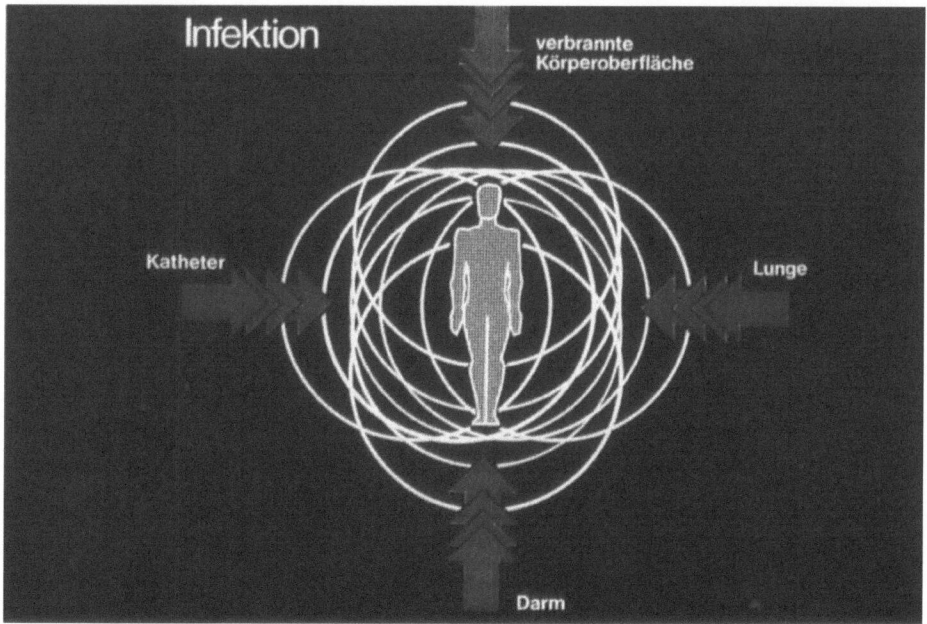

Abb. 1. Infektionsquellen beim Brandverletzten

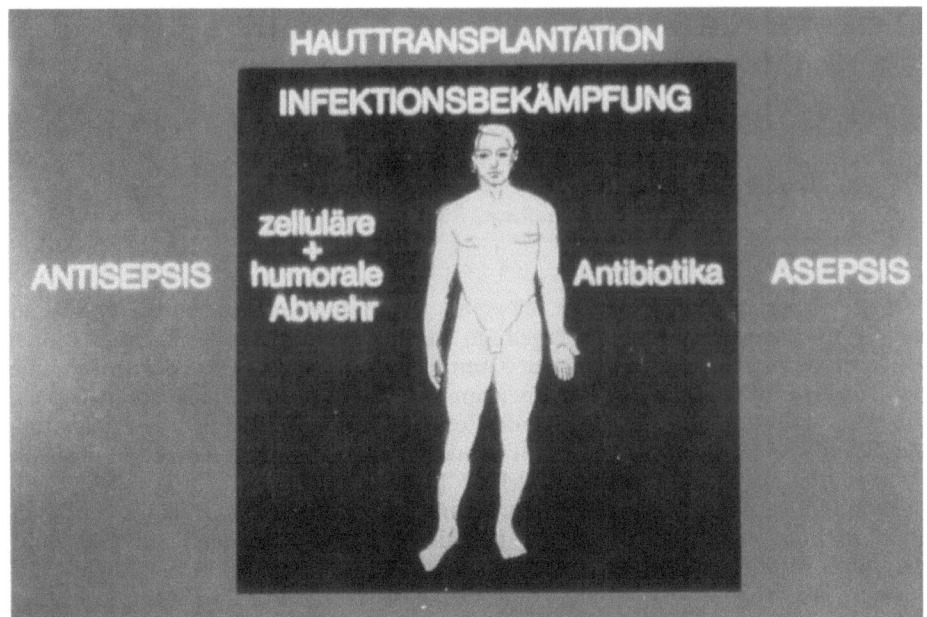

Abb. 2. Infektionsverhütung und -bekämpfung beim Brandverletzten

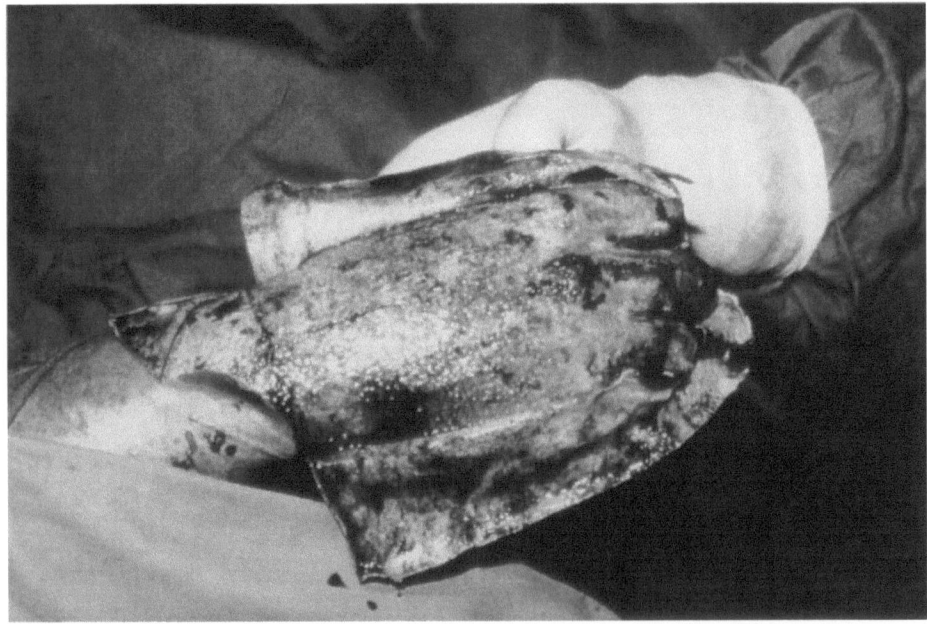

Abb. 3. Die mit PVP-Jod behandelte Nekrose hat sich demarkiert und kann leicht entfernt werden

Tabelle 1. Die Forderungen, die man an ein Oberflächenbehandlungsmittel stellen muß:

1. Es muß atoxisch sein und darf keine Verschiebung des Stoffwechsels verursachen.
2. Es muß ein gutes mikrobizides Spektrum haben.
3. Es muß in den Wundschorf eindringen und ihn durchdringen.
4. Es muß gegenüber dem überlebenden und proliferierenden Gewebe inaktiv sein.
5. Es darf nicht antigen sein.
6. Es darf nicht zu einer bakteriellen Resistenz führen.
7. Es soll eine gerbende Wirkung haben.

Tabelle 2. Unterschiedliche Definitionen zum Timing des chirurgischen Vorgehens bei Verbrennungen in der Literatur

Begriff	Definition
prompt eschar excision	keine genaue Zeitangabe
early excision	1.–10. Tag post trauma (72 Std. nach Aufnahme) Excision von 20–25% KOF
early major burn wound excision	2.–7. Tag post trauma Excision des größten Teils der 3.-grad. Verbrennungen
early massive excision	72 Std. nach Aufnahme Excision aller 3.-grad. Verbrennungen
early staged excision	3.–5. Tag post trauma schrittweise Excision von je 20% KOF
late excision	später als 7. Tag post trauma
serial debridement	tägliche Bäder
konservativ	regelmäßig scharfes Debridement Transplantation auf Granulationen

chenbehandlungsmittel gestellten Anforderungen sind aus der Tabelle 1 zu ersehen. Eingehende Qualitätsprüfungen nach der Methode von Brentano haben eine sehr gute Keimreduktion auf den Wunden nachgewiesen und statistische Erhebungen und Publikationen im amerikanischen Schrifttum haben eindeutig gezeigt, daß nach Wiedereinführung einer routinemäßigen Oberflächentherapie die Sterblichkeit durch Septikämie deutlich zurückgegangen ist, so daß man dieser Therapie eine hohe Wertigkeit beimessen muß.

In der BG-Unfallklinik Ludwigshafen wird seit vielen Jahren das PVP-Jod erfolgreich eingesetzt. Bei diesem Präparat kommt zu der lokal mikrobiziden Wirkung ein gerbender Effekt hinzu, der die thermisch zerstörte Haut in eine derbe, braun pigmentierte Nekrose mit guter Abgrenzung zum vitalen Gewebe überführt (Abb. 3). Trotzdem bleibt eine gute Tiefenwirkung erhalten, da das Jod auch dicke Nekrosen in antiseptisch wirksamer Konzentration penetriert. Damit wird eine planmäßige und schrittweise Nekrektomie unter Berücksichtigung des Allgemeinzustandes des Patienten möglich. Zweitgradige Verbrennungen heilen unter der schützenden Nekrose, die nach vollständiger Epithelisation der Wunde abgestoßen wird.

Der Anstieg des Jodserumspiegels unter PVP-Jodtherapie zeigt deutlich die gute Penetration des Jods durch die Nekrose. Es finden sich dabei keine wesentlichen Unterschiede bei den Schilddrüsenhormonen und TSH im Vergleich zu polytraumatisierten Patienten, die nicht mit PVP-Jod behandelt wurden. Eine Stoffwechselentgleisung im Sinne einer Thyreotoxikose konnte bei über 2500 Brandverletzten nicht beobachtet werden.

Das Timing der Nekrektomie ist nach wie vor ein Diskussionsthema. Die Nomenklatur ist nicht einheitlich und in der Definition häufig unklar und mißverständlich. Die in Tabelle 2 aufgeführten Beispiele untermauern diese Kritik. Die Verwirrung wird noch gesteigert, wenn Mortalitätsstatistiken der 60er Jahre mit solchen aus den späten 80er und 90er Jahren verglichen werden, um den positiven Effekt der frühzeitigen Nekrektomie zu beweisen. Dabei bleiben wesentliche Faktoren wie die rasante Weiterentwicklung der Intensivmedizin in den letzten 2 Jahrzehnten unberücksichtigt, und damit sind solche Vergleiche nicht statthaft. In die Überlegungen zur Wahl des Zeitpunkts der chirurgischen Intervention ist auch der Verlauf der Ödemausbildung und Rückresorption mit einzubeziehen. Auf dem Höhepunkt des Verbrennungsödems ist eine Operation sicherlich riskanter als nach Einsetzen der Rückresorption mit beginnender Stabilisierung des Kreislaufs (Abb. 4).

Zur Einteilung des chirurgischen Vorgehens im Hinblick auf die Wahl des Zeitpunkts schlagen wir ein Schema vor, das sich an dem Verlauf des Verbrennungsödems orientiert. Abbildung 5 zeigt eine Uhr, deren Ziffern die Tage nach dem Verbrennungstrauma bedeuten. Daneben stellt eine Kurve den Gewichtsverlauf beim Brandverletzten in den Tagen 1–12 nach dem Trauma dar.

Die Primärexcision ist nun die partielle oder totale Nekrektomie vor dem Höhepunkt der Ödemeinlagerung, d.h. in den ersten 24–72 Stunden nach dem Unfall (Abb. 6, Tab. 3).

Die postprimäre Excision erstreckt sich bei bereits beginnender Ödemausschwemmung vom 3.–9. Tag nach dem Unfall (Abb. 7, Tab. 4).

Von einer sekundären Excision sprechen wir, wenn nach etwa 10 Tagen nach weitgehender Ausschwemmung des Ödems bei einer gemischten Verbrennung verbliebene Nekrosen an umschriebenen Bereichen excidiert werden müssen (Abb. 8, Tab. 5).

Die postprimäre Excision zwischen dem 3. und 9. Tag bei beginnender Ausschwemmung des Ödems ist das bevorzugte Timing in Ludwigshafen. Seit Eröffnung

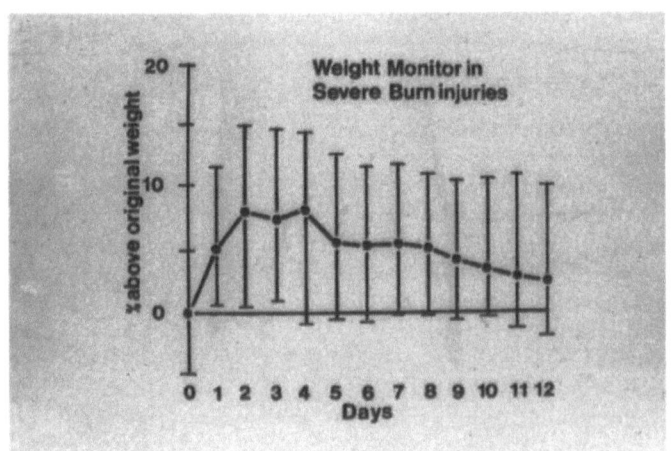

Abb. 4. Entwicklung des Körpergewichts nach schweren Verbrennungen, unter Infusionstherapie (Ludwigshafener Formel)

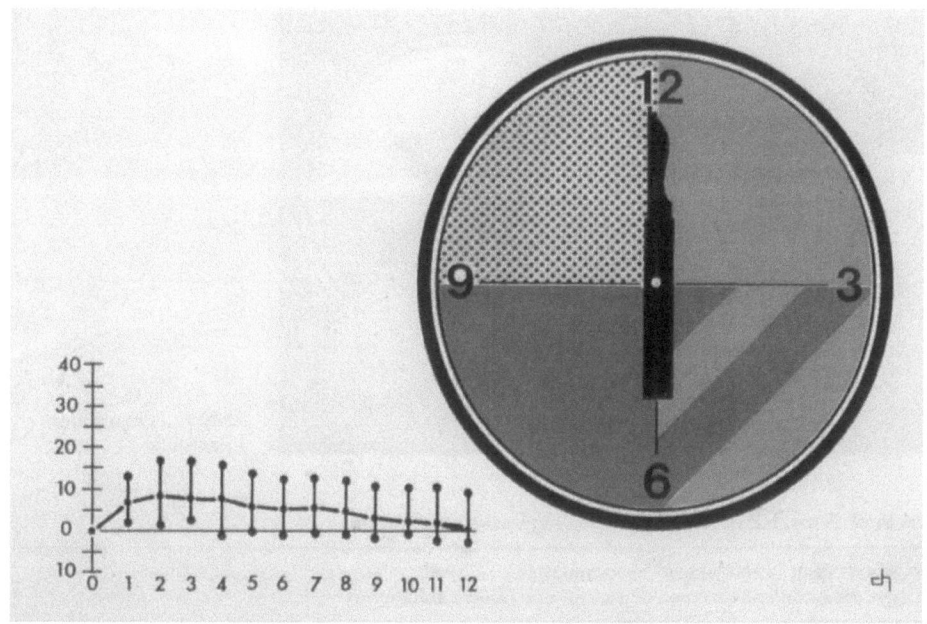

Abb. 5. Vorschlag zur Einteilung des chirurgischen Vorgehens (Erklärung im Text)

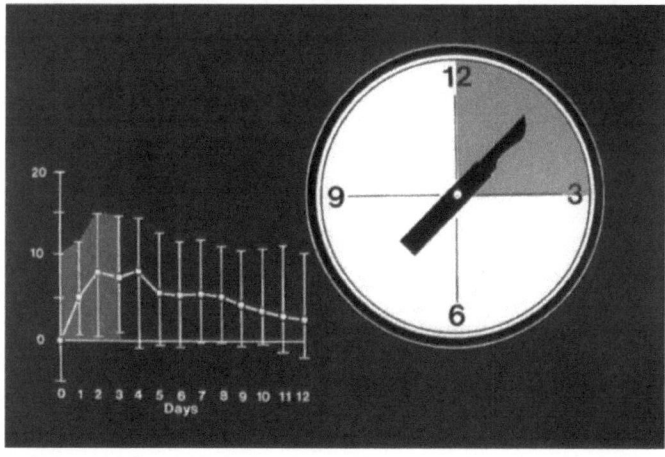

Abb. 6. Primäre Excision

Tabelle 3. Primäre Excision (partiell/total) 24–72 Std. nach dem Trauma

- Verbrennungen der Ohren
- Verbrennungen der Augenlider
- Verbrennungen der Hände
- Elektroverbrennungen
- Kontaktverbrennungen
- Verbrennungen <10% Körperoberfläche
- hohes Lebensalter des Patienten

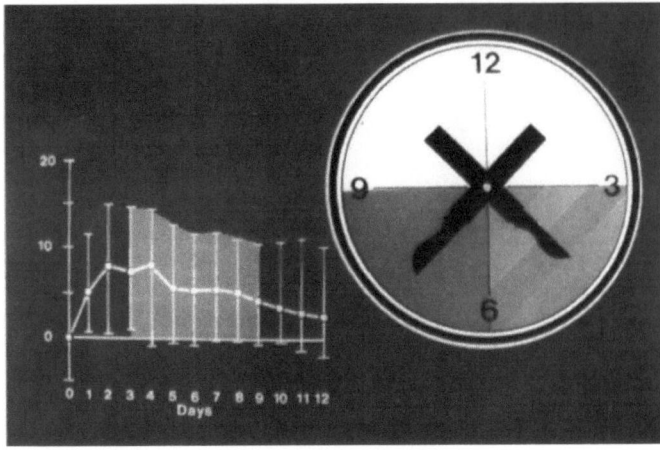

Abb. 7. Postprimäre Excision

Tabelle 4. Postprimäre Excision (3.–9. Tag nach dem Trauma)

- drittgradige, großflächige Verbrennungen
- bevorzugtes Verfahren in der BG Klinik Ludwigshafen

der Station im Jahre 1969 haben wir die thermisch zerstörte Haut immer so früh wie möglich epifascial entfernt, wobei uns die Nekrektomie auf dem Höhepunkt der Ödemeinlagerung keine Vorteile hinsichtlich der Mortalität gegenüber der postprimären aufgezeigt hat. Bei ausgedehnten Verbrennungen können höchstens 25–30% der Körperoberfläche in einer Sitzung excidiert werden. Der nächste Eingriff kann dann meist erst nach 2 Tagen durchgeführt werden, ein dritter erst nach weiteren 2 Tagen, so daß bis zur vollständigen Nekrektomie 1 Woche vergangen ist. Damit ist ein wesentlicher Zeitgewinn durch primäre Excision im Vergleich zur postprimären Excision nicht gegeben, wohl aber ein erhöhtes Operationsrisiko.

Die Technik der Excision wird ebenfalls diskutiert. Die tangentiale Technik wenden wir nur bei umschriebenen Verletzungen oder dort an, wo es um die Erhaltung der Form geht, wie z. B. bei der Verbrennung der weiblichen Brust. Im überwiegenden Teil der Fälle ist bei schweren Verbrennungen die epifasciale Excision vorzuziehen. Die Nekrektomie kann dabei mit dem Skalpell, dem elektrischen Messer oder mit dem Laserskalpell durchgeführt werden. Die Arbeit mit dem CO_2-Laser ist zwar zeitaufwendig, dafür spart man Zeit bei der Blutstillung (Abb. 9a, b) und der Blutverlust ist insgesamt nur halb so groß wie bei den konventionellen Verfahren. Eine Schädigung des Empfängerbettes tritt nach unseren ausgedehnten histologischen Untersuchungen nicht ein.

Zur temporären Deckung, die wir bei ausgedehnten Nekrektomien zur Versorgung der Wundfläche immer durchführen, stehen uns mehrere Möglichkeiten zur Verfügung (Tabelle 6). Wir bevorzugen die menschliche Fremdhaut und haben bereits 1970 eine Hautbank in Ludwigshafen etabliert. Wir möchten hervorheben, daß unsere Studie zum Thema typisierte Fremdhaut hinsichtlich der Verweildauer wesentliche Vorteile erbracht hat. Gerade durch ausgedehnte Nekrektomien hat das

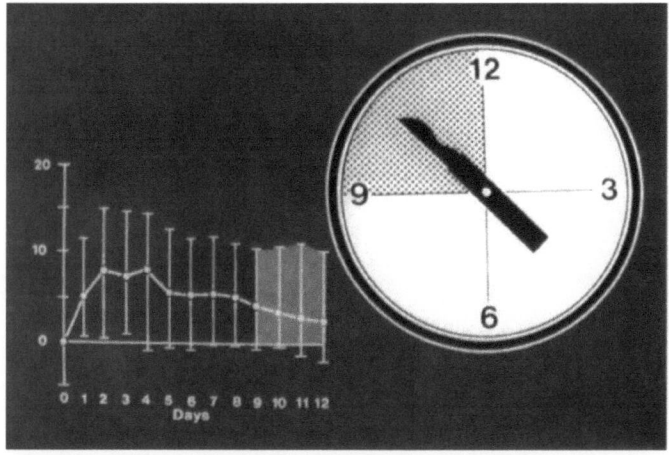

Abb. 8. Sekundäre Excision

Tabelle 5. Sekundäre Excision (10. Tag nach Trauma und später)

- hauptsächlich zweitgradige Verbrennungen
- primär inoperable Patienten

Tabelle 6. Temporäre Wunddeckung beim Brandverletzten

- Allotransplantat (Homotransplantat) typisiert/nicht typisiert/frisch/ tiefgefroren/konserviert
- Xenotransplantat (Heterotransplantat) Schweinehaut
- „Kunsthaut", Folien etc.

Tabelle 7. Endgültige Wunddeckung beim Brandverletzten

- Spalthaut
    Meshgraft
    Sheetgraft
- Vollhaut
- Lappenplastik (gestielt/frei)
- gemischte autochtone-allogene Verfahren „Chinesische Methode" sog. Overgrafting
- Zellkulturen (Keratinozyten)

Problem der temporären Deckung besondere Bedeutung gewonnen. Für die Epithelzüchtung werden etwa 3 Wochen benötigt. Somit muß auch bei dieser Technik eine temporäre Deckung erfolgen. Die Epithelzüchtung hat jedoch noch keinen überzeugenden Erfolg erbracht, so daß man geneigt ist, der Gewebetypisierung erneut Bedeutung beizumessen, da sich hier die Verweildauer in günstigen Fällen auf 6 Wochen belaufen kann. Es läßt sich histologisch eine deutliche Gefäßeinsprossung in die Transplantate nachweisen, was im Hinblick auf die Verringerung der Keiminvasion von der Oberfläche her sicher positiv bewertet werden muß.

Die Routine bei der definitiven Deckung wird in 1. Linie das Spalthauttransplantat, gemesht oder ungemesht, sein (Tabelle 7). Die chinesische Methode hat sich in Deutschland nicht durchgesetzt. Jedoch wird man dem Overgrafting bei einem Meshgrafttransplantat von 1:6 einen positiven Effekt nicht absprechen können. Bei

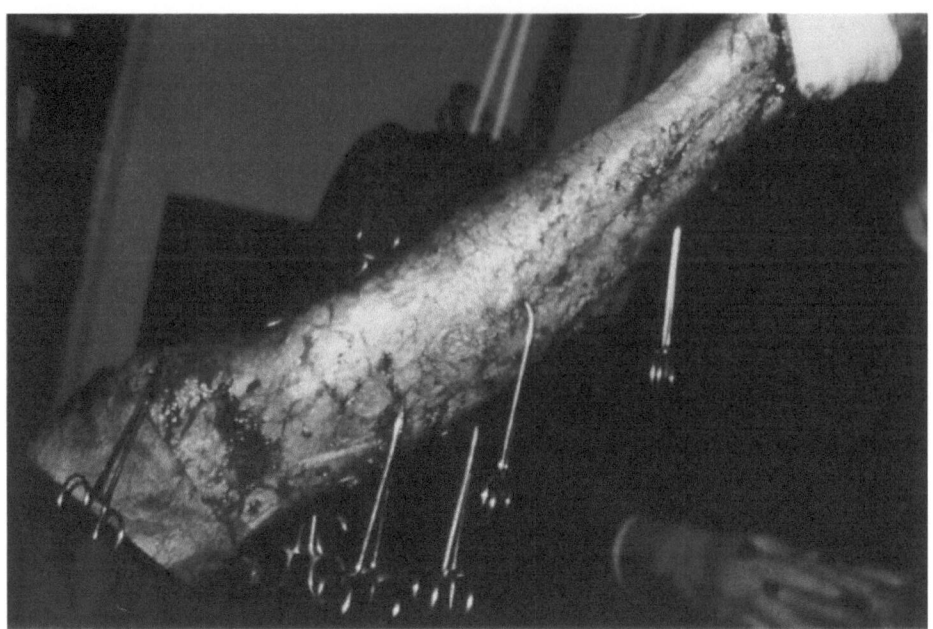

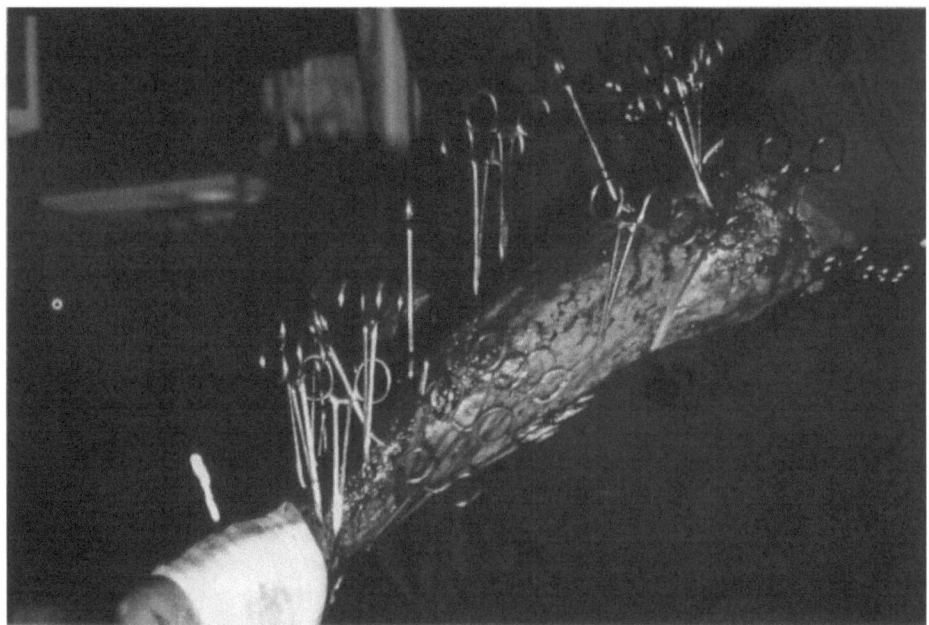

Abb. 9a, b. Die Nektrektomie mit dem CO_2-Laser (**a**) ist wesentlich unblutiger als die mit dem Skalpell (**b**)

dem jetzigen Stand der Transplantationstechnik wird es wesentlich sein, daß man die Spenderbezirke mehrmals benutzen kann. Aus der Literatur geht hervor, daß hier mehrere Ansätze vorhanden sind, die es ermöglichen, bei limitierten Spenderbezirken eine erneute Entnahme von Spalthaut bereits vor dem 10. Tag durchzuführen.

Wir werden nur nach eingehenden Statistiken, die eine glaubhafte Aussage über die Mortalität unterschiedlicher Techniken ergeben, unser Timing bei der Nekrektomie erneut evaluieren. Solange dies nicht der Fall ist, sollte man den großzügigen Empfehlungen mancher Publikationen nicht kritiklos folgen. Die temporäre Defektdeckung ist nach wie vor ein Problem, besonders wenn immer ausgedehntere Excisionen durchgeführt werden. Wenn wir nicht in der Lage sind, diese Wunden schnell mit Eigenhaut zu decken, so tauschen wir nur die eine Wunde gegen eine andere ein.

Für die Verfasser:
Prof. Dr. Dr. P. R. Zellner
Atos Praxisklinik Heidelberg
Bismarckstraße 9–15
D-69115 Heidelberg

Hyperbaric oxygen therapy in the treatment of thermal burns

P. E. Cianci

Brookside Hospital, San Pablo

Introduction

The use of hyperbaric oxygen as an adjunct in the treatment of thermal injury is considered controversial. It is frequently condemned as being too dangerous and/or too expensive for routine use. A comprehensive review of the world literature fails to support these conclusions. A significant body of data suggest it may be of great benefit and its utilization can favorably affect outcome relative to length of hospital stay, surgical procedures, reduction of infection, and mortality.

Background

Hyperbaric oxygen therapy is an outgrowth of Naval diving programs throughout the world whereby divers suffering from decompression illness ("the bends") were treated by being pressurized in large, metal, hyperbaric chambers.

The use of hyperbaric oxygen therapy in the treatment of thermal burns began serendipitously in 1965, when Ikeda and Wada noted more rapid healing of second-degree burns in a group of coal miners that were being treated for carbon monoxide poisoning [41]. They followed this observation with a series of experiments that demonstrated a reduction of edema and improved healing in animal studies [22]. The Japanese experience [21–23, 41, 42] stimulated interest in other countries, and a series of uncontrolled clinical reports began to accumulate, all of which demonstrated favorable results [28, 40]. In 1970, Gruber, [15] working at the U.S. Biophysics Laboratory at the Edgewood Arsenal in Maryland, U.S.A., devised a series of experiments in which rats were placed in a hyperbaric chamber while breathing 100% oxygen at sea level and at the pressure equivalent of 2 and 3 atmospheres, respectively. He demonstrated that the area subjacent to a third-degree burn was hypoxic when compared to normal skin and that the tissue oxygen tension in these areas could only be raised by oxygen administered at pressure. This important study suggested that hyperbaric oxygen therapy could have a direct effect on the pathophysiology of the burn wound (Fig. 1).

Pathophysiology

In order to understand the rationale for therapy, it is necessary to review the physiology of the thermal injury. The burn wound is a complex and dynamic injury characterized by a central zone of coagulation surrounded by an area of stasis bordered by an area of erythema. The zone of coagulation or complete capillary

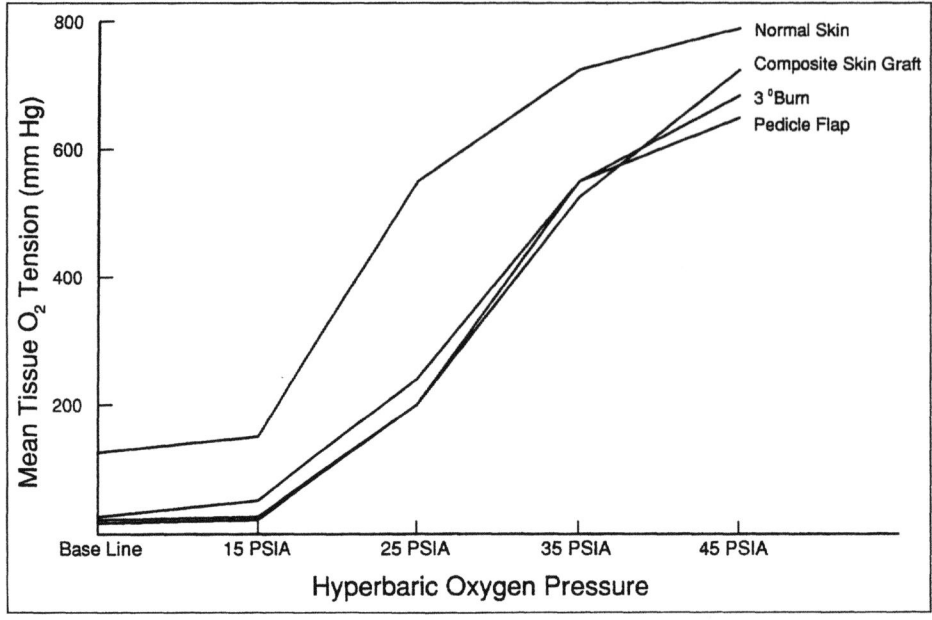

Fig. 1. Mean oxygen tension of normal skin and various hypoxic tissue as a function of hyperbaric oxygen pressure. Note: Oxygen tension rises in burned skin only with increasing pressure. (By permission [15].)

occlusion may progress by a factor of 10 during the first 48 h after injury. Ischemic necrosis quickly follows. Hematologic changes, including platelet microthrombi and hemoconcentration, occur in the post-capillary venules. Edema formation is rapid in the area of injury, but also develops in distant, uninjured tissue. There are also changes occurring in the distal microvasculature where red cell aggregation, white cell adhesion to the endothelium of venular walls, and platelet thromboemboli occur [6]. "This progressive ischemic process, when set in motion, may extend damage dramatically during the early days after injury [19]." The ongoing tissue damage seen in thermal injury is due to the failure of surrounding tissue to supply borderline cells with oxygen and nutrients necessary to sustain viability [3]. The impediment to circulation below the injury leads to dessication of the wound as fluid cannot be supplied via the thrombosed or obstructed capillaries. Topical agents may reduce but cannot prevent dessication of the burn wound and the inexorable progression to deeper layers.

Infection

Susceptibility to infection is greatly increased owing to the loss of the integumentary barrier to bacterial invasion, the ideal substrate present in the burn wound, and the compromised or obstructed microvasculature which prevents humoral and cellular elements from reaching injured tissue. Additionally, the immune system is seriously affected, demonstrating decreased levels of immunoglobulins and serious perturbations of PMN function [1, 2, 12, 35]. These include disorders of chemotaxis, phagocytosis, and diminished killing ability. These functions greatly increase morbidity and mortality; infection remains the leading cause of death from burns. Regeneration cannot take place until equilibrium is reached; hence, healing is retarded. Prolongation of the healing process may lead to excessive scarring. Hypertrophic scars are seen in 4% of cases taking 10 days to heal, 14% of those taking 14 days or less, and in 28% of cases taking 21 days or more. In those cases taking over 21 days, scarring may be as high as 40% of cases [11]. Therapy of burns, then, should be directed towards minimizing edema, protecting the microvasculature, preserving marginally viable tissue, enhancing host defenses, and providing the essential substrate necessary to sustain viability and fight infection.

Experimental evidence

A significant body of animal data support the efficacy of hyperbaric oxygen in the treatment of thermal injury. Ikeda noted a reduction of edema in burned rabbits [22]. Ketchum in 1967 reported an improvement in healing time and reduced infection in an animal model [25]. He later demonstrated dramatic improvement in the microvasculature of burned rats treated with hyperbaric oxygen therapy [26]. In 1974, Hartwig and colleagues [18] working in Germany reported very similar findings and additionally noted less inflammatory response in those animals that had been treated with hyperbaric oxygen. He suggested at that time that hyperbaric oxygen therapy might be a useful adjunct to the technique of early tangential excision. Wells and Hilton [44], in a carefully controlled and designed experiment, reported a marked decrease in extravasation of fluid in a series of dogs with 40% flame burns (Fig. 2). The effect was clearly related to oxygen and not simply increased pressure. They also

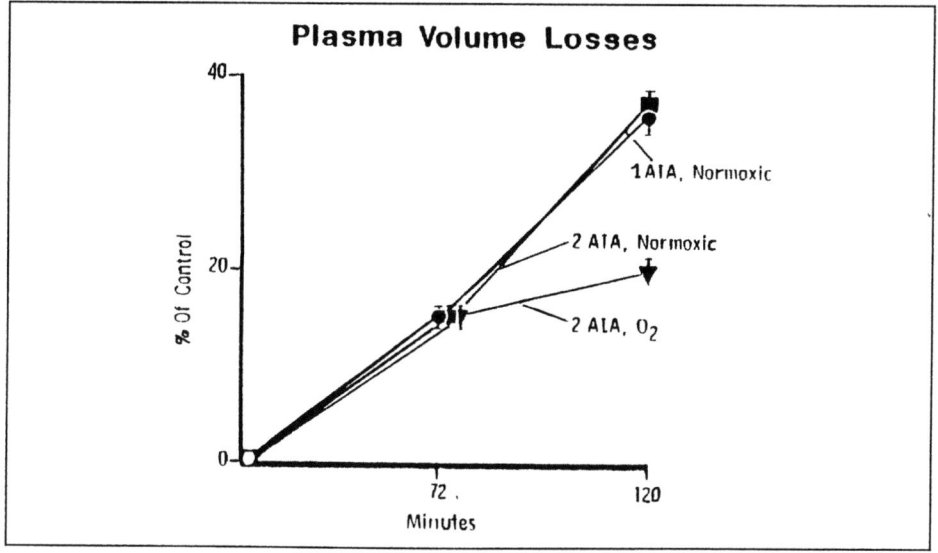

Fig. 2. Plasma volume losses after burn in untreated animals (1 ATA, normoxic), animals exposed to hyperbaric oxygen (2 ATA, O_2) and to pressure alone (2 ATA, normoxic). (By permission [44].)

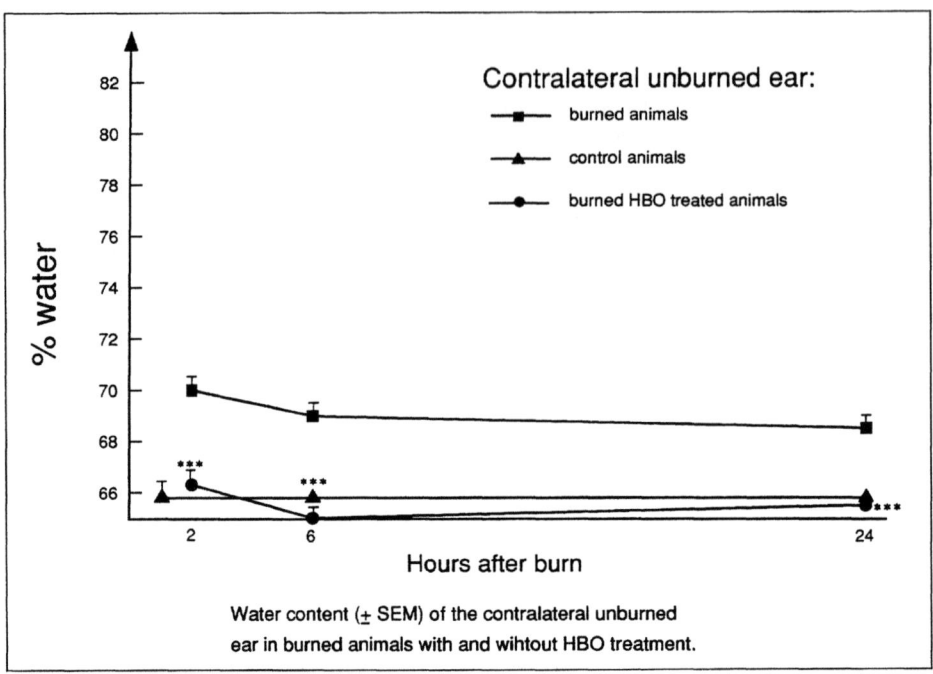

Fig. 3. Water content (±SEM) of the contralateral unburned ear in burned animals with and without HBO treatment. (By permission [34].)

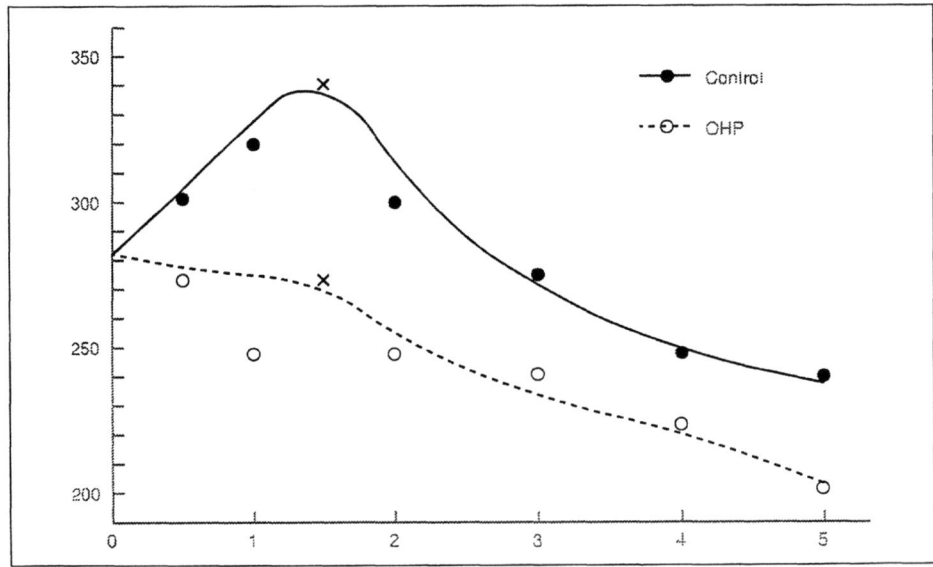

Fig. 4. Average wound surface area (mm^2). Experimental third-degree burns increase over time in control animals. HBO-treated animals showed shrinkage of wounds. (Modified from Kaiser by permission [24].)

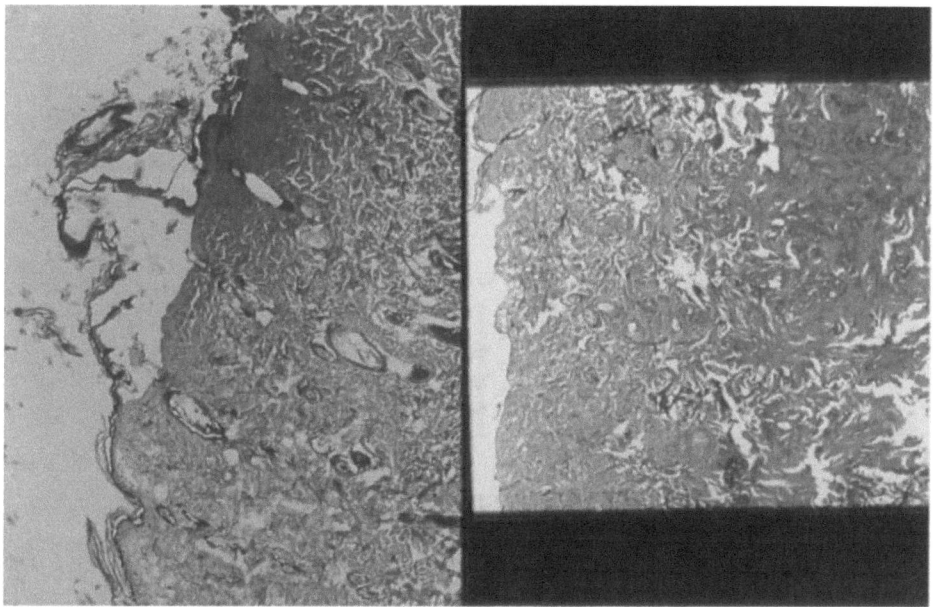

Fig. 5. Biopsy of experimental partial thickness burns at 5 days. A) HBO-treated animals showed preservation of the dermal elements. B) Nontreated animals showed coagulation necrosis.

reported a reduction in hemoconcentration and improved cardiac output in treated dogs. Nylander [34] in a well-accepted animal model showed that hyperbaric oxygen therapy reduced the generalized edema associated with burn injury (Fig. 3). Kaiser and colleagues from Germany have recently demonstrated a significant reduction of subcutaneous edema in burned animals treated with hyperbaric oxygen therapy. He has reported a progression of the burn wound in control animals while the hyperbaric-treated animals showed a decrease in wound size (Fig. 4) [24]. Korn and colleagues [27], in 1977, showed an early return of capillary patency in the hyperbaric-treated animals using an India ink technique. He also demonstrated survival of the dermal elements and more rapid epithelialization from these regenerative sites. He suggested that the decreased dessication of the wound he observed was felt to be a function of subjacent capillary integrity noted in the hyperbaric-treated animals. Saunders and colleagues [37] from the University of Chicago have recently reported preservation of the microcirculation and collagen quality in a similar experiment. Perrins failed to show a beneficial effect in a scald wound in a pig model treated with hyperbaric oxygen [36]. Niccole [32], in 1977, reported that hyperbaric oxygen offered no advantage over topical agents in controlling wound bacterial counts. He proposed that hyperbaric oxygen alone acted as a mild antiseptic. His data, however, supported the observation of improved healing of partial thickness injury noted by earlier investigators. Stewart [38, 39] and colleagues have shown preservation of adenosine triphosphate (ATP) in areas subjacent to partial thickness in burns in hyperbaric-treated rats. Biopsies of the wounded animals showed progression to full thickness injury in the controls, whereas preservation of the dermal elements and capillary patency was observed in the hyperbaric-treated animals (Fig. 5). These

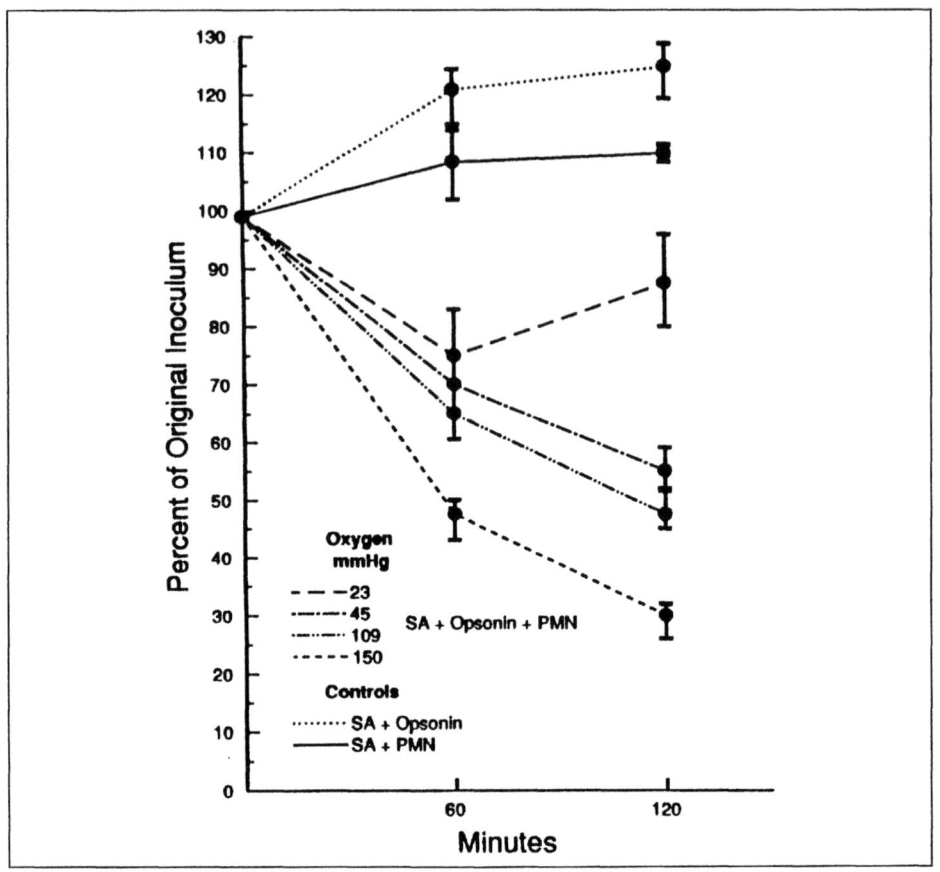

Fig. 6. Phagocytic killing of Staphylococcus aureus under different oxygen tension. (From Mader [29].)

studies relate directly to the preservation of energy sources for the sodium pump and white cell killing. Failure of the sodium pump is felt to be a major factor in the ballooning of the endothelial cells that occurs after burn injury and subsequent massive fluid losses [4]. Both groups in Stewart's study received identical treatment with topical antibiotic agents. Bleser [5], in 1973, in a large controlled series from France reported a reduction of burn shock and a fourfold increased survival in 30% burned animals vs. controls.

Reduction of polymorphonuclear cell killing ability in hypoxic tissue has been well documented by Hohn et al. [20]. The ability of hyperbaric oxygen to elevate tissue oxygen tension and the enhancement of PMN killing in an O_2-enriched animal model as demonstrated by Mader [29] suggests that this may be an additional benefit of hyperbaric oxygen (Fig. 6). Thus, the overwhelming evidence in a large number of controlled animal studies suggests that hyperbaric oxygen reduces edema, preserves the microcirculation, prevents conversion of partial to full thickness injury, preserves the sodium pump by maintaining high levels of ATP, improves survival, and, though not yet proven, may well enhance PMN killing in the burn scenario.

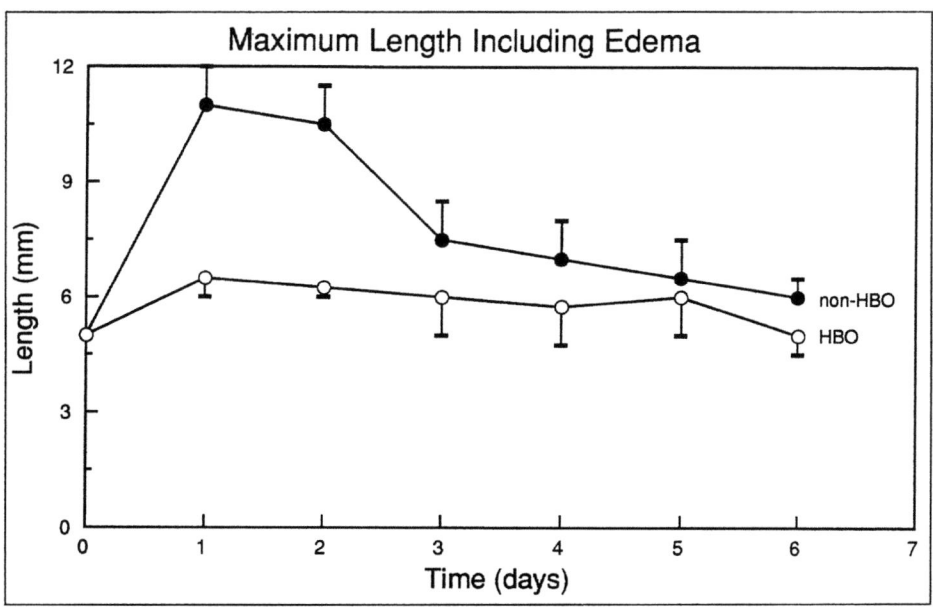

Fig. 7. Maximum length (including oedema adjacent to the wound) (Mean ±SD) of u.v.-irradiated and HBO-treated u.v.-irradiated blister wounds as a function of time. The value on day 0 is approximately the diameter of the suction cup used to create the blister ($p < 0.05$). (From Hammerlund [16].)

Human experience

Beginning with Wada in 1965, and continuing with Ikeda [21–23, 41, 42], Lamy [28], and Tabor [40], reports of clinical series began to accumulate. In 1974, Hart [17] reported a controlled, randomized series showing a reduction of fluid requirements, faster healing, and reduced mortality when his patients were compared to national controls in the U.S. National Burn Information Exchange standards. Waisbren [43], in 1982, reported a reduction in renal function, a decrease in circulating WBC's, and an increase in positive blood cultures in a retrospective series of patients who had received hyperbaric oxygen therapy at his burn center. He stated, however, that he could demonstrate neither a salutary nor deleterious effect; however, his data showed a 75% decrease in the need for grafting in the hyperbaric-treated group. Grossman and colleagues [13, 14, 45] in California have amassed a very large clinical series showing improved healing, reduced hospital stay, and reduced mortality. Merola and colleagues [31] in Italy, in 1978, reported a randomized study showing faster healing of partial thickness burns in 37 patients treated with hyperbaric oxygen vs. 37 untreated controls. Niu and his associates [33] from the Naval burn center in Taiwan have recently reported a very large clinical series showing a statistically significant reduction in mortality in 266 seriously burned patients who had received adjunctive hyperbaric oxygen therapy when compared to 609 control patients who did not receive this additional modality of therapy. Infection was reduced in the hyperbaric oxygen-treated patients. Hammerlund and colleagues [16] have reported a reduction of edema and wound exudation in a carefully controlled series of human

Table 1. Comparison of factors in HBO and Non-HBO groups in patients with 18–39% TBSA burns.

Variable	HBO ($n = 8$)	Control ($n = 12$)	
Age (yr)			
Average	29.5	30.9	
Range	16–47	18–42	$p<0.57$ NS
Standard deviation	9.6	8.5	
Total body surface burn (%)			
Average	24.0	25.8	
Range	20–33	18–39	$p<0.91$ NS
Standard deviation	4.3	7.6	
Full-thickness injury			
Average	5.2	5.6	
Range	0–18	0–20	$p<0.96$ NS
Standard deviation	6.1	6.2	
Surgeries			
Average	1.3	1.7	
Range	0–2	0–3	$p<0.42$ NS
Standard deviation	0.88	1.2	
Days hospitalized			
Average	20.8	33.0	
Range	16–33	16–58	$p<0.012$*
Standard deviation	6.7	13.1	
Cost of burn care			
Average	$44,838	$55,650	
Range	$27,600–$75,500	$21,500–$98,700	$p<0.47$ NS
Standard deviation	$9,200	$11,300	

NS, Not significant.
* $p<0.012$, significant (Mann-Whitney U-test).

volunteers with ultraviolet-irradiated blister wounds (Fig. 7). Cianci has shown a significant reduction in length of hospital stay in burns of up to 39% of total body surface area [9] (Table 1). Additionally, this group has reported a reduction in the need for surgery in burns of 40–80%, including grafting, tracheostomies, escharotomies, etc. [8] (Table 2). Hyperbaric oxygen-treated patients in this study represented an additional advantage of $95,000 savings per case. In a retrospective, blinded review a 25% reduction in resuscitative fluid administration and a statistically significant reduction in maximum weight gain was noted in the hyperbaric oxygen-treated group vs. controls [7]. Maxwell and colleagues in 1991 reported a small controlled series showing a reduction of surgery, resuscitative weight gain, intensive care days, total hospitalization time, cost of hospitalization, and wound sepsis in the hyperbaric-treated patients [30].

Table 2. Comparison of factors in HBO and Non-HBO groups in patients with 40–80% TBSA burns.

	HBO ($n=6$)	Control ($n=6$)	
Age (yr)			
Average	25.7 ± 4.6	33.3 ± 9.8	$p=0.064$ NS
Range	20–31	14–42	
Total body surface burn			
Average	61.7 ± 18.6%	49.8 ± 8.5%	$p=0.309$ NS
Range	40–80%	40–60%	
Full-thickness injury			
Average	23.7 ± 21.3%	23.5 ± 15.5%	$p=0.818$ NS
Range	0–50%	7–50%	
Surgeries			
Average	3.7 ± 2.6	8.0 ± 3.4	$p=0.041$
Range	0–6	3–12	
Days hospitalized			
Average	65.3 ± 23.4	111.0 ± 57.7	$p=0.132$ NS
Range	42–95	47–184	
Cost			
Average	$185,000 ± 90,500	$292,300 ± 184,300	$p=0.309$ NS
Range	$110,000 – 318,000	$114,000 – 602,000	
HBO cost			
Average	$15,500 ± 10,000 [a]		
	$ 4,800 – 25,900		

[a] Eight percent of the total hospital bill.
NS = not significant.

Discussion

The work of Hohn and colleagues [20] has demonstrated that hypoxic tissue is susceptible to infection; conversely, correction of hypoxic tissue increases resistance to bacterial invasion. Hyperbaric oxygen can attack this problem directly, preserving levels of ATP, maintaining the microcirculation, and reducing or preventing edema formation, thus allowing better exchange of tissue gases and immune systems. White cell killing is known to be diminished in burns. Enhancement of white cell killing ability is proportional to rising levels of tissue oxygen tensions [29] (Mader figure). This increase in tissue O_2 levels in the burn injury should enhance host resistance. More rapid healing of partial thickness injury reduces the risk of bacterial invasion.

Summary

Current data demonstrate that hyperbaric oxygen therapy when used as an adjunct in a comprehensive program of burn care can significantly improve morbidity and mortality, reduce length of hospital stay, and lessen the need for surgery. It has been demonstrated to be safe in the hands of those thoroughly trained in rendering hyperbaric oxygen in the critical care setting and with appropriate monitoring precautions. Careful patient selection and screening are mandatory. The use of hyperbaric oxygen as an adjunct in the treatment of thermal injury merits consideration.

References

1. Alexander JW, Wilson D (1970) Neutrophil dysfunction and sepsis in burn injury. Surg Gynec Obstet 130:431
2. Alexander JW, Meakins JL (1972) A physiological basis for the development of opportunistic infections in man. Annals of Surgery 176:273
3. Arturson G (1980) Pathophysiology of the burn wound. Ann Chir Gynaecol 66:178–190
4. Arturson G (1985) The pathophysiology of severe thermal injury. J Burn Care Rehab 6(2):129–146
5. Bleser F, Benichoux R (1973) Experimental surgery: the treatment of severe burns with hyperbaric oxygen. J Chir (Paris) 106:281–290
6. Boykin JV, Eriksson E, Pittman RN (1980) In vivo microcirculation of a scald burn and the progression of postburn dermal ischemia. Plast and Recon Surg 66:191–198
7. Cianci P, Lueders H, Lee H, Shapiro R, Green B, Williams C (1988) Hyperbaric oxygen and burn fluid requirements: observations in 16 patients with 40–80% TBSA burns. Undersea Biomedical Research Suppl 15:14
8. Cianci P, Lueders H, Lee H, Shapiro R, Sexton J, Williams C, Green B (1988) Adjunctive hyperbaric oxygen reduces the need for surgery in 40–80% burns. J Hyperbar Med 3:97–101
9. Cianci P, Lueders H, Lee H, Shapiro RL, Sexton J, Williams C, Sato R (1989) Adjunctive hyperbaric oxygen therapy reduces length of hospitalization in thermal burns. J Burn Care Rehab 10:432–435
10. Cianci P, Williams C, Lueders H, Lee H, Shapiro R, Sexton J, Sato R (1990) Adjunctive hyperbaric oxygen in the treatment of thermal burns: an economic analysis. J Burn Care Rehab 11:140–143
11. Deitch E, Wheelahan T, Rose M, Clothier J, Cotter J (1983) Hypertrophic burn scars: analysis of variables. J Trauma 23:895–898
12. Grogan JB (1976) Altered neutrophil phagocytic function in burn patients. J Trauma 16:734
13. Grossman AR (1978) Hyperbaric oxygen in the treatment of burns. Ann Plast Surg 1:163–171
14. Grossman AR, Grossman AJ (1982) Update on hyperbaric oxygen and treatment of burns. HBO Review 3:51–59
15. Gruber RP, Brinkley B, Amato JJ, Mendelson JA (1970) Hyperbaric oxygen and pedicle flaps, skin grafts, and burns. Plast and Recon Surg 45:24–30
16. Hammarlund C, Svedman C, Svedman P (1991) Hyperbaric oxygen treatment of healthy volunteers with u.v.-irradiated blister wounds. Burns 17(4):296–301
17. Hart GB, O'Reilly RR, Broussard ND, Cave RH, Goodman DB, Yanda RL (1974) Treatment of burns with hyperbaric oxygen. Surg Gynec Obstet 139:693–696
18. Hartwig VJ, Kirste G (1974) Experimentelle Untersuchungen über die Revaskularisierung von Verbrennungswunden unter hyperbarer Sauerstofftherapie. Zbl Chir 99:1112–1117
19. Heggers JP, Robson MC, Zachary LS (1980) Thromboxane inhibitors for the prevention of progressive dermal ischemia due to the thermal injury. J Burn Care Rehab 6:466–468
20. Hohn DC, MacKay RD, Halliday B, Hunt TK (1976) Effect of oxygen tension on the microbicidal function of leukocytes in wounds and in vitro. Surgical Forum 27:18–20
21. Ikeda K, Ajiki H, Kamiyama I, Wada J (1967) Clinical application of oxygen hyperbaric treatment. Geka (Japan) 29:1279
22. Ikeda K, Ajiki H, Nagao H, Karino K, Sugh S, Iwa T, Wada J (1970) Experimental and clinical use of hyperbaric oxygen in burns. In: Wada J, Iwa T (eds) Proceedings of the Fourth International Congress on Hyperbaric Medicine. Tokyo: Igaku Shoin Ltd., pp 370–380
23. Iwa T. Discussion. In: Brown JW, Cox BG (eds) Proceedings of the Third International Conference on Hyperbaric Medicine. Washington, DC; National Academy of Science–National Research Council. Publication No. 4, 1966
24. Kaiser VW, Schnaidt U, Lieth H von der (1989) Auswirkungen hyperbaren Sauerstoffes auf die frische Brandwunde. Handchir Mikrochir Plast Chir 21:158–163
25. Ketchum SA, Zubrin JR, Thomas AN, Hall AD (1967) Effect of hyperbaric oxygen on small first, second and third degree burns. Surgical Forum 18:65–67
26. Ketchum SA, Thomas AN, Hall AD (1970) Angiographic studies of the effect of hyperbaric oxygen on burn wound revascularization. In: Wada J, Iwa T (eds) Proceedings of the Fourth International Congress on Hyperbaric Medicine. Tokyo: Igaku Shoin Ltd., pp 388–394

27. Korn HN, Wheeler ES, Miller TA (1977) Effect of hyperbaric oxygen on second-degree burn wound healing. Arch Surg 112:732–737
28. Lamy ML, Hanquet MM (1970) Application opportunity for OHP in a general hospital – a two years experience with a monoplace hyperbaric oxygen chamber. In: Wada J, Iwa T (eds) Proceedings of the Fourth International Congress on Hyperbaric Medicine. Tokyo: Igaku Shoin, Ltd., pp 517–522
29. Mader JT, Brown GL, Guckian JC, Wells CH, Reinarz JA (1980) A mechanism for the amelioration of hyperbaric oxygen of experimental staphylococcal osteomyelitis in rabbits. J Inf Disease 142:915–922
30. Maxwell G, Meites H, Silverstein P (1991) Cost effectiveness of hyperbaric oxygen therapy in burn care. Winter Symposium on Baromedicine, 1991
31. Merola L, Piscatelli F (1978) Considerations on the use of HBO in the treatment of burns. Ann Med Nav 83:515–526
32. Niccole MW, Thornton JW, Danet RT, Bartlett RH, Tavis MJ (1977) Hyperbaric oxygen in burn management: a controlled study. Surgery 82:727–733
33. Niu AKC, Yang C, Lee HC, Chen SH, Chang LP (1987) Burns treated with adjunctive hyperbaric oxygen therapy: a comparative study in humans. J Hyper Med 2:75–86
34. Nylander G, Nordstrom H, Eriksson E (1984) Effects of hyperbaric oxygen on oedema formation after a scald burn. Burns 10:193–196
35. Ogle CK, Alexander JW, Nagy H, Wood S, Palkert D, Carey M, Ogle JD, Warden JD (1990) A long-term study and correlation of lymphocyte and neutrophil function in the patient with burns. J Burn Care Rehab 11(2):105–111
36. Perrins DJD (1970) Failed attempt to limit tissue destruction in scalds of pig's skin with hyperbaric oxygen. In: Wada J, Iwa T (eds) Proceedings of the Fourth International Congress on Hyperbaric Medicine. Tokyo: Igaku Shoin Ltd., pp 381–387
37. Saunders J, Fritz E, Ko F, Bi C, Gottlieb L, Krizek T (1989) The effects of hyperbaric oxygen on dermal ischemia following thermal injury. In: Proceedings of the American Burn Association p 58
38. Stewart RJ, Yamaguchi KT, Cianci PE, Knost PM, Samadani BA, Mason SW, Roshdieh B (1988) Effects of hyperbaric oxygen on adenosine triphosphate in thermally injured skin. Surgical Forum 39:87–90
39. Stewart RJ, Yamaguchi KT, Cianci PE, Mason SW, Roshdieh BB, Dabbass N (1989) Burn wound levels of ATP after exposure to elevated levels of oxygen. In: Proceedings of the American Burn Association p 67
40. Tabor CG (1967) Hyperbaric oxygenation in the treatment of burns of less than forty percent. Korean J Int Med
41. Wada J, Ikeda T, Kamata K, Ebuoka M (1965) Oxygen hyperbaric treatment for carbon monoxide poisoning and severe burn in coal mine (Hokutanyubari) gas explosion. Igakunoaymi (Japan), pp 54–68
42. Wada J, Ikeda K, Kagaya H, Ajiki H (1966) Oxygen hyperbaric treatment and severe burn. Jap Med J 13:2203
43. Waisbren BA, Schultz D, Collentine G, Banaszak E, Stern M (1982) Hyperbaric oxygen in severe burns. Burns 8:176–179
44. Wells CH, Hilton JG (1977) Effects of hyperbaric oxygen on post-burn plasma extravasation. In: Davis JC, Hunt TK (eds) Hyperbaric Oxygen Therapy, Bethesda: Undersea Medical Society, Inc., pp 259–265
45. Wiseman DH, Grossman AR (1985) Hyperbaric oxygen in the treatment of burns. Crit Care Clin 2:129–145

Author's address:
Paul Cianci, M.D., F.A.C.P.
Professor of Medicine
University of California, Davis
Director, Hyperbaric Medicine
Brookside Hospital
2000 Vale Road
San Pablo, CA 94806, USA

Die Antibiotikatherapie beim Brandverletzten

G. Germann

Abteilung für plastische Chirurgie und Verbrennungskrankheiten BG, Universitätsklinik Bergmannsheil, Bochum

Antibiotikatherapie bei Brandverletzten

Infektionen bilden auch heute noch das größte Mortalitätsrisiko schwerverbrannter Patienten. Die Letalität systemischer Infektionen erreicht 50–75%, bei Patienten mit Lungenversagen steigt die Letalität einer infektiösen pulmonalen Komplikation auf 90% [20, 21]. Gerade der Brandverletzte mit seinem in der Postaggressionsphase erheblich eingeschränkten Immunsystem ist den Gefahren einer bakteriellen Besiedelung besonders ausgesetzt. Bei dieser massiven Infektionsgefährdung der Patienten steht die Verhütung infektiöser Komplikationen neben einer frühzeitigen stabilen Hautdeckung im Mittelpunkt der therapeutischen Strategie. Auch der Einsatz antimikrobiell wirksamer Substanzen ist fester Bestandteil dieses Konzepts. Die Grenzen zwischen Indikation und Kontraindikation eines Antibiotikaeinsatzes erscheinen allerdings oft verwaschen, so daß die Rolle der Antibiotikatherapie beim Brandverletzten eine kritische Würdigung verdient [11, 20, 22, 29, 41].

Antibiotika stellen in der modernen Intensivmedizin einen wesentlichen Faktor in der Bekämpfung und möglicherweise auch in der Prophylaxe schwerer Infektionen dar, sind aber auch die größten Kostenfaktoren. Neben den unzweifelhaften Segnungen, welche die Entwicklung der Antibiotika für viele Patienten bedeutet hat, birgt der unkritische Einsatz der potenten Substanzen gerade im Intensivbereich ein nicht zu unterschätzendes Gefahrenmoment. Dazu gehören neben den enormen Kostensteigerungen vor allem der Selektionsdruck mit der Entwicklung multiresistenter Problemkeime, aber auch die klinischen Situationen, in denen die Gabe hochwirksamer Antibiotika die physiologische Situation des Patienten rapide verschlechtern kann [8, 9, 17, 20, 37, 41].

Seit Einführung der Antibiotika in die klinische Routine ist die Heilungsrate bakterieller Infektionen deutlich gestiegen. Auch die Überlebensrate schwerbrandverletzter Patienten konnte dadurch in den frühen 50er Jahren deutlich gesteigert werden (Abb. 1). Dagegen konnte die Letalitätsrate septischer Patienten in den letzten 15 Jahren durch den Einsatz potenter Breitspektrumantibiotika nicht signifikant gesenkt werden. So findet sich z.B. bei polytraumatisierten Patienten, bei Brandverletzten ist dies noch nicht untersucht, eine deutliche negative Korrelation zwischen häufigem Präparatewechsel, Länge der AB Therapie und schlechtem "outcome". In Blutkulturen dieser Patienten wurden durch ein wirksames Antibiotikum in vielen Fällen der eliminierte Keim nur durch einen resistenten Stamm ersetzt [3, 22].

. Diese Überlegungen müssen in ein antimikrobielles Therapiekonzept einbezogen werden (Tabelle 1). Ein wichtiger Platz gebührt der Infketionsverhütung. Dazu gehören vor allem strikte Hygiene am Patienten, die Unterbrechung der Kontaminationswege (Abb. 2), die Anwendung prophylaktischer Physiotherapie wie Atemgymna-

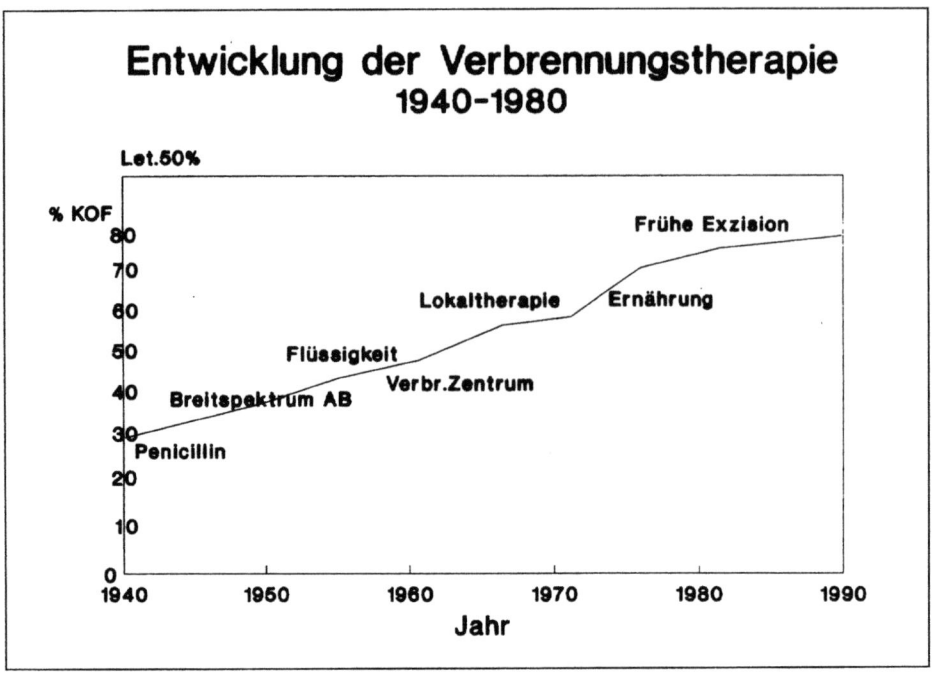

Abb. 1. Entwicklung der Brandverletzungsbehandlung und der Sterblichkeit von 1930–1980. Die Letalität konnte jeweils mit einer wichtigen Ergänzung der therapeutischen Konzepte gesenkt werden

Tabelle 1. Antimikrobielles Therapiekonzept

– strikte Hygiene
– Unterbrechung der Kontaminationswege
– prophylaktische Physiotherapie
– topische Therapie
– kritischer Antibiotika-Einsatz
– keine „Schrotschußtherapie"

stik, Lagerungswechsel etc. und eine frühe enterale Ernährung. Hygienische Defizite sind durch Antibiotika *nicht* auszumerzen und auch die erwähnten prophylaktischen Maßnahmen wie Atemgymnastik oder Physiotherapie sind in der Verhütung einer Pneumonie sicher höher einzuschätzen als der Einsatz von Antibiotika. Vielfach wird in einem „Beschuß" der Patienten mit möglichst vielen, einander komplementierenden Substanzen, der Weg gesehen, eine infektiöse Komplikation zu verhindern. Leider gelingt dies, auch bei Einsatz bester Präparate nur bedingt. Eine solche breitgestreute „Schrotschußtherapie" ist in jedem Falle abzulehnen [6, 11, 15, 17, 33].

Es gilt daher rationale Kriterien für den Einsatz von Antibiotika im Intensivbereich und hier speziell im Gebiet der Brandverletzung zu erarbeiten. Wo ist der

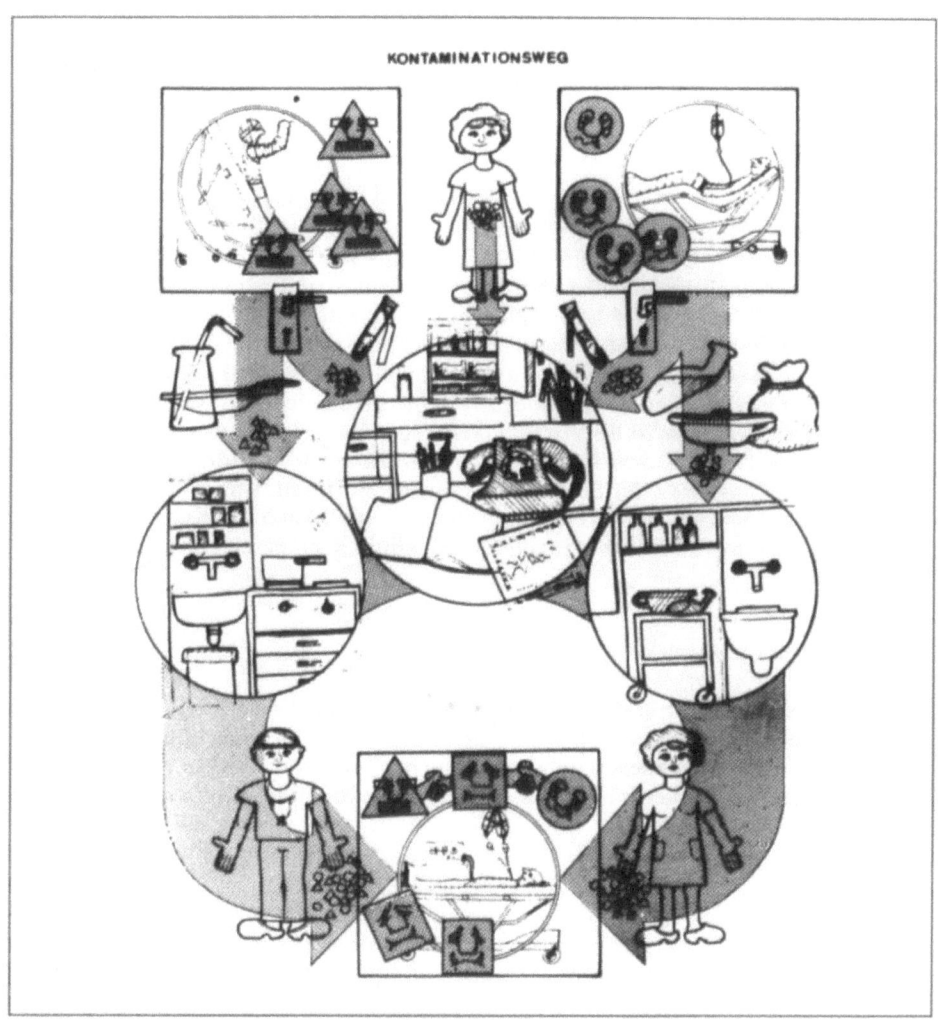

Abb. 2. Mögliche Kontaminationswege im Krankenhaus

Einsatz sinnvoll, wann ist er fragwürdig und in welchen Fällen sollte der Einsatz von Antibiotika unterbleiben?

Dazu steht heute neben den klassischen Penicillinen und Cephalosporinen der 1. und 2. Generation ein kaum noch zu überblickendes Arsenal von Antibiotika und Antimykotika zur Verfügung. Ungeachtet der getroffenen Präparateauswahl ist die Beschränkung auf ein bestimmtes Sortiment zu empfehlen, das natürlich im Bedarfsfall ergänzt werden kann. Dies hat mehrere Vorteile:

1. Alle Mitarbeiter sind mit Spektrum, Dosierung und eventuellen Nebenwirkungen vertraut.
2. Weniger erfahrene Mitarbeiter haben ein Gerüst, auf das sie sich stützen können.

3. Kosteneinsparung und Lagerungskapazität machen die Beschränkung auf ein festes Sortiment nötig.

Penicilline

Bei den Penicillinen spielen die „alten" Benzyl- und Phenoxypenicilline nur noch bei Streptokkoken-Phlegmonen eine klinisch bedeutsame Rolle. In der Behandlung klinisch bedeutsamer Staphylokokkeninfekten sind sie von Penicillinase-festen Penicillinen wie Flucloxacillin abgelöst worden. Ampicillin und seine Derivate werden heute in der Regel wegen der hohen Allergisierungsrate fast ausschließlich in Saftform bei Kindern angewendet, obwohl weiterhin eine sehr gute Wirksamkeit gegenüber Enterokokken besteht. Die Acylureidopenicilline (Mezlocillin, Azlocillin, Piperacillin und Apalcillin) sind im gramnegativen Spektrum deutlich besser wirksam als alle Vorgänger, haben dafür an Wirksamkeit gegenüber Staphylococcus aureus eingebüßt. Diesem Nachteil wurde versucht durch die Kombination mit Enzymhemmern wie Clavulansäure oder Sulbactam entgegenzuwirken, was sich in einer deutlich gesteigerten klinischen Wirksamkeit niederschlug. Auch die Kombination von Acylureidopenicillin und Flucloxacillin wird klinisch eingesetzt [31, 34, 37] (Tabelle 2, Tabelle 3).

Cephalosporine - β Lactame

Die Cephalosporine der ersten Generation (z.B. Cefazolin) erlitten ein ähnliches Schicksal wie die Penicilline, obwohl kein spürbarer Wirkungsverlust feststellbar war. Sie wurden durch neuere Cephalosporine mit breiterem Wirkungsspektrum im gramnegativen Bereich verdrängt (u.a. Cefotiam, Cefamandol, Cefoxitin). Die dritte

Tabelle 2. Penicilline

Generic	Handelsname
Penicillin „G"	Penicillin G
Flucloxacillin	Staphylex
Ampicillin	Binotal
Amoxycillin	Amoxypen
Mezlocillin	Baypen
Azlocillin	Securopen
Piperacillin	Pipril
Apalcillin	Lumota

Tabelle 3. Kombinationspräparate

Generic	Handelsname
Clavulansäure + Amoxycillin	Augmentan
Sulbactam + Ampicillin	Unacid
Piperacillin + Flucloxacillin	Fluxapril
Sulbactam + ?	Combactam

Generation der Cephalosporine (Cefotaxim, Ceftriaxon, Ceftozoxim, Cefmenoxin) brachte dann den Durchbruch zum echten „Breitbandantibiotikum", büßte aber deutlich im grampositiven Spektrum ein, so daß nur eine mäßige klinische Wirksamkeit gegenüber Staphylokokken verblieb [31, 34].

Einige Cephalosporine weisen eine überdurchschnittliche Wirksamkeit gegen Pseudomonas aeruginosa species auf und haben sich als Reserveantibiotika bei vital bedrohlichen Infektionen bewährt (Ceftazidim, Cefsulodin). In dieser Gruppe sind auch noch zwei andere β-Lactamantibiotika zu erwähnen, das Imipenem und das Aztreonam. Das Imipenem gehört zu den Substanzen mit dem breitesten mikrobiologischen Spektrum; das Aztreonam bleibt schweren gramnegativen Infektionen vor allem mit multiresistenten Enterobacteriaceae und Pseudomonaden vorbehalten (Tabelle 4).

Aminoglykoside

Die Aminoglykoside gehören auch heute noch zum festen Repertoire der Antibiotikatherapie. Die bekannten Nebenwirkungen auf Niere und Gehörsystem lassen sich durch ein pharmakologisches Drug Monitoring weitgehend ausschließen. In den angloamerikanischen Ländern wird dennoch durchweg, trotz der bekannten Risiken, höher dosiert. Der Schwerpunkt der Substanzgruppe liegt in einer guten Wirksamkeit gegen gramnegative Enterobakterien und vor allem Pseudomonaden. Das Spektrum ist für alle Mitglieder der Gruppe vergleichbar, allerdings wird Substanzen wie Tobramycin und Amikacin eine Reservefunktion bei nachgewiesener Gentamycinresistenz zugeschrieben. Klinisch werden immer wieder wechselnde Resistenzmuster gefunden, so auch Gentamycinsensibilität bei Amikacinresistenz. Besonders geeignet sind die Aminoglykoside in der Kombinationstherapie mit β-Lactamen [31, 34] (Tabelle 5).

Tetracycline

Tetracycline spielen in der Infektionsbekämpfung auf Brandverletztenstationen nur noch in Ausnahmefällen eine Rolle.

Chinolone

Stark hervorgetreten sind in den letzten Jahren die Vertreter der Chinolone. In Deutschland kommen vor allem Ofloxacin und Ciprofloxacin zum Zug. Das Cipro-

Tabelle 4. Cephalosporine

Generic	Handelsname
Cefazolin	Gramaxin
Cefamandol	Mandokef
Cefoxitin	Mefoxitin
Cefotaxim	Claforan
Cefmenoxin	Tacef
Cefsulodin	Pseudocef
Ceftazidim	Fortum

Tabelle 5. Aminoglykoside

Generic	Handelsname
Gentamycin	Refobacin
Sisomycin	Extramycin
Netilmycin	Certomycin
Tobramycin	Gernebcin
Amikazin	Biklin

Tabelle 6. Chinolone

Generic	Handelsname
Enoxazin	Gyramid
Ofloxacin	Tarivid
Ciprofloxacin	Ciprobay

Tabelle 8. Antimykotika

Generic	Handelsname
Amphotericin B	Amphotericin B
Muconazol	Daktar
Fluconazol	Diflucan
Flucytosin	Ancotil

Tabelle 7. Wichtige sonstige Antibiotika

Generic	Handelsname
Cilastatin + Imipenem	Zienam
Aztreonam	Azactam
Teicoplanin	Targocid
Vancomycin	Vancomycin

floxacin zeichnet sich durch die größte in vitro-Aktivität aus, klinisch erscheinen die Substanzen vergleichbar. Die Vorteile der Chinolone liegen im breiten Spektrum, sowohl im gram-negativen, wie im grampositiven Bereich. Die Resistenzquote bei Pseudomonaden liegt zwischen 6–15%. Hervorzuheben ist die große therapeutische Breite dieser Stoffgruppe [27, 31, 34, 36] (Tabelle 6).

Sonstige

Einige Antibiotika haben sich durch ihre speziellen Wirkungsbereiche eine Sonderstellung erworben, die sie zu unverzichtbaren Waffen im therapeutischen Arsenal macht. Hierzu gehören vor allem Vancomycin und Teicoplanin. Vancomycin hat sich als Reservesubstanz bei multiresistenten Staphylokokken über viele Jahre bewährt. Die Erfahrungen mit Teicoplanin sind prinzipiell ebenfalls gut, allerdings gab es in der klinischen Einführungsphase noch Dosierungsprobleme. Die Indikation sind Staphylokokkeninfektionen bei nachgewiesener Multiresistenz der Erreger oder Verdacht auf Therapieversager mit herkömmlichen Staphylokokken-wirksamen Präparaten [8, 31, 34]. (Tabelle 7)

Antimykotika

Moderne Antimykotika stammen vorwiegend aus der Stoffgruppe der Azole. Wichtigste Vertreter sind Miconazol, Ketoconazol und Fluconazol. Sie sind gegen die gängigsten nosokomialen Pilzinfektionen wirksam, allerdings zeigt nur Miconazol eine ausreichende Wirksamkeit gegen Aspergillus. Die Azole gelten als weniger toxisch als die Polyene, deren wichtigste i.v. applizierbarer Vertreter das Amphotericin B ist. Es weist auch eine hervorragende Wirksamkeit gegen Aspergillus auf und wird bei Verdacht auf Candida Sepsis aus Gründen der Dosisreduktion häufig mit Fluocytosin kombiniert. Derzeit wird ein in Liposomen verkapseltes Amphotericin B in die Klinik eingeführt, was eine erheblich geringere Toxizität bei gleicher Wirksamkeit aufweisen soll [11, 31, 34] (Tabelle 8).

Erregerspektrum

Zwei Keime beherrschen auch heute noch das Spektrum der isolierten Erreger, Pseudomonaden und Staphylokokken. Allerdings treten mittlerweile auch vermehrt Wundinfektionen und Sepsisfälle durch andere gramnegative Problemkeime wie Enterobacter cloacae, Klebsiella, E. coli, Acinetobacter, Serratia species aber auch ganz vereinzelt Providencia und Morganellen auf. Probleme bereiten niemals die „normalen" Angehörigen dieser Gattung, sondern die multiresistenten Problemstämme. Die Multiresistenz ist zumeist Folge des „iatrogenen" Selektionsdrucks durch Antibiotikatherapie. Gerade Pseudomonas species, Enterobacter calcoaceticus und resistente Staphylokokken können so bis zu ihrer „Enttarnung" verheerende Folgen auslösen. Diese Gratwanderung zwischen der Bekämpfung dieser Problemkeime und ihrer „hausgemachten" Züchtung durch großzügigsten, unkritischen Antibiotikaeinsatz kann bei geringer Abweichung vom richtigen Weg zu erheblichen Infektionsproblemen auf einer Brandstation führen [6, 7, 16, 18, 28, 30, 32, 40].

Bedingt durch das Keimspektrum und die oft kritische klinische Lage der Patienten finden auf Brandstationen zunehmend primär Antibiotika der jüngeren Generationen Verwendung, oft allerdings bei durchaus noch vorhandener Wirksamkeit älterer Präparate. Hier wird die prinzipiell gegebene Indikation zur antibiotischen Therapie, vielfach aus Unsicherheit und der Absicht Fehler zu vermeiden, sofort mit dem Einsatz des neuesten Präparates beantwortet. Gerade aber der unkritische Einsatz von Breitspektrumantibiotika unter Vernachlässigung der auch hier vorhandenen Lücken leistet der Entwicklung multiresistenter Species Vorschub. Es erscheint durchaus sinnvoll, bei kontinuierlich dokumentiertem Erreger- und Resistenzprofil einer Station, eine Stufentherapie anzustreben, die primär Präparate mit einem schmaleren Spektrum benutzt, bei Bedarf auf Kombinationstherapie, und erst bei klinischem Mißerfolg oder nachgewiesener Resistenz auf eine der Reservesubstanzen zurückgreift [4, 11, 28, 30].

Unter Beachtung dieser Risiken und Probleme gilt es also zu evaluieren, wann welcher Einsatz von Antibiotika bei Brandverletzten sinnvoll und medizinisch begründbar ist und in welchen klinischen Situationen eine Anwendung von Antibiotika eher nachteilige Effekte hat.

Prophylaxe

Eine antibiotische Prophylaxe wurde und wird sicher auch noch in vielen Abteilungen gerne bei Inhalationstrauma (IHT) und schweren Verbrennungen durchgeführt. Die Wirksamkeit eines solchen Regimes ist aber eher mit Skepsis zu betrachten, da eine Senkung der Infektionsrate, beim IHT z.B. der Pneumonie, bzw. eine Senkung der Mortalität nicht erreicht werden konnte. An einem eigenen Kollektiv von ca. 280 Patienten aus den Jahren 1988–1990 wurde durch prophylaktische Antibiotika in Relation zu einer historischen, aber vergleichbaren Gruppe, keine Verbesserung der Infektionsrate erzielt.

Eine generelle Antibiotikaprophylaxe bei Schwerverbrannten ist abzulehnen. Die Immunsuppression des Schwerverbrannten ist durch die Gabe selektionierender Antibiotika nicht zu verbessern. Eine Besiedlung der Wunde ist möglicherweise aufzuhalten, aber auch mit den breitesten Antibiotika in Höchstdosen nicht ganz zu verhindern. Hier erscheint das Risiko des Selektionsdrucks deutlich höher als der Nutzen für den Patienten [5].

Auch bei Leichtverbrannten in ambulanter Behandlung hat der prophylaktische Einsatz von Antibiotika nicht zu einer Reduktion der Wundinfektionsrate geführt [5, 38]. Auch die experimentelle Infusion unter die Verbrennungsnekrose hat keine Kontaminationsminderung erzielen können [27].

Erfolgversprechender erscheint der Einsatz prophylaktischer Antibiotika bei der Spalthauttransplantation nach tangentieller oder epifaszialer Exzision. Bei der operativen Nekrosenabtragung kommt es zu einer nachweisbaren Bakteriämie. Die Rate der konsekutiven Septikämien wird durch eine prophylaktische Antibiotikagabe jedoch nicht reduziert [4, 25]. Allerdings zeigen die Arbeiten Krizeks einen deutlichen Zusammenhang zwischen quantitativer Keimbesiedelung und „take rate" der Transplantate. Die Angehrate von Spalthauttransplantaten nimmt bei einer Keimdichte $>10^6$ rapide ab. Gelingt es mit einer Antibiotikaapplikation die Kontamination der Wunde zu senken, ist eine kurzfristige perioperative Prophylaxe sicher indiziert, da ohne das Risiko einer Resistenzentwicklung, eine Verbesserung der klinischen Situation des Patienten erreicht werden kann. Je höher die „take rate" desto eher kommt der Organismus des Patienten aus dem katabolen, hypermetabolen Zustand heraus. Die Wahl des Antibiotikums richtet sich nach der Resistenzprüfung; liegt diese noch nicht vor, muß eine „kalkulierte Prophylaxe" durchgeführt werden [9, 20].

Aus der Tatsache der Operation folgert aber nicht zwangsläufig die Indikation zur Prophylaxe. Eine früh durchgeführte tangentielle Exzision mit nachfolgender Deckung durch autologe Haut bedarf in der Primärphase der Verbrennung keiner antibiotischen Prophylaxe. Überschreitet der Operationszeitpunkt dagegen die ersten 5 Tage und liegen deutliche Zeichen einer Wundkontamination vor, erscheint die perioperative Prophylaxe sinnvoll.

Die Selektive Darm Dekontamination (SDD) mit schwer bzw. nicht resorbierbaren Antibiotika hat in ausgewählten Kollektiven die Morbidität z.B. im Sinne der Rate pulmonaler Infekte deutlich senken können aber keine signifikante Senkung der Mortalität erzielt. Mit einem ähnlichen Regime konnte im eigenen Kollektiv durch die Übernahme der „Swish & swallow" Prophylaxe gegen Pilze eine deutliche Verringerung der Pilzinfektionen mit einer Senkung der Inzidenz letaler Pilzseptikämien erzielt werden. Ob die antibakterielle SDD ähnliche Effekte bei homogenen Kollektiven schwerverbrannter Patienten hat, bleibt abzuwarten, erscheint aber nicht unwahrscheinlich; erste Studien zeigen eine Minderung der Translokation, aber keine Verbesserung der Überlebensrate [1, 12, 13, 19, 31, 35].

Die intratracheale Prophylaxe mit einem Aminoglykosid hat sich in den Händen einzelner bewährt. Im Bereich der Verbrennung liegen nur wenige Berichte über die Effizienz dieser Methode vor [37].

Therapie

Eine klare Indikation zur Antibiotikatherapie liegt bei jeder gesicherten Infektion des Brandverletzten vor. Angesichts der erheblichen Immunsuppression und der damit verbundenen Infektanfälligkeit muß aber erwogen werden, ob nicht auch bei ausreichend begründetem Verdacht eine Therapie erfolgen sollte [11, 16, 28, 30, 41].

Hierbei sollte in Betracht gezogen werden, daß die alleinige Entwicklung von Temperaturen nach einem Verbrennungstrauma keinen Beweis für eine bakterielle Infektion darstellt. Das Verbrennungstrauma an sich ist mit dem Vorhandensein großer avitaler Gewebebezirke und der Freisetzung einer Unzahl von Mediatoren, von denen etliche pyrogene Wirkungen haben (IL2, IL6), verbunden. Die physiologische Reaktion ist ausreichend für die Entwicklung einer erhöhten Temperatur, die zusätzlich Ausdruck der hypermetabolen Situation des Patienten ist, die wiederum durch die gleichen Mediatorensysteme gesteuert wird. Eine Infektion z.B. am ersten Tag post Trauma nur aufgrund der erhöhten Körpertemperatur anzunehmen ist daher sicherlich falsch und leistet wiederum dem Prinzip der „schädlichen Prophylaxe" Vorschub.

Der Verdacht auf eine bakterielle Infektion sollte daher klinisch erhärtet sein. Oft taucht in diesem Zusammenhang der Begriff der „burn wound sepsis" auf. Der Begriff ist verwirrend und wird je nach Benutzer mit unterschiedlichen Inhalten verbunden. Prinzipiell wird damit der Zustand einer infizierten Brandwunde und nicht gleichzeitig eine generalisierte Infektion im Sinne einer „Sepsis" beschrieben. Ob eine infizierte, schmierig belegte Brandwunde einer systemischen Antibiotika Therapie bedarf, kann nicht ex juvantibus beantwortet werden. Sicherlich hängt dies vom Ausmaß der infizierten Fläche, dem Zustand des Patienten, dem Verbrennungsausmaß insgesamt und der schon exzidierten und gedeckten Fläche ab. Wichtige Erkenntnisse liefert zudem die quantitative Wundbiopsie [21]. Einen Patienten mit ca. 50% verbrannter KOF, der noch Restdefekte von ca. 5% hat und schon mobilisiert ist, wird man wegen einer schmierigen Wunde kaum systemisch mit einem Antibiotikum behandeln, einen Patienten mit 40% KOF, der, aus welchen Gründen auch immer, nicht frühzeitig operiert werden konnte und Zeichen einer Allgemeininfektion aufweist, wird man sicher therapieren müssen [2, 10, 11, 16, 30].

Die antimikrobielle Therapie der Brandwunde wird primär also aus topischen oder chirurgischen Methoden bestehen und nur bei Verdacht auf eine Allgemeininfektion mit Fokus Brandwunde einer systemischen Therapie bedürfen. Hilfreich sind in diesem Zusammenhang quantitative Wundbiopsien, um den Invasionsgrad und die Spezies der invadierenden Bakterien abschätzen zu können [11, 15, 16, 20, 25, 28, 30, 33].

Eine spezielle Situation stellt der Starkstromverbrannte dar. Hier kommt es auch bei konsequentem seriellem Débridement zur Entwicklung fokaler Muskelnekrosen. Selbst bei sauberster Verbandtechnik ist eine Kontamination noch weniger vermeidbar als bei „normalen" Brandwunden. Hier ist eine antibiotische Therapie/Prophylaxe im Zweifel früher angebracht als in anderen Situationen, da auch die vitale Gefährdung des Patienten durch das Vorhandensein von Restmuskelnekrosen höher einzustufen ist. Pulmonale Infektionen sind eine eindeutige Indikation für eine Antibiotika Therapie. Schwierig ist hier nur die Diagnose. Röntgenbilder sind, gerade bei Patienten mit IHT, nicht eindeutig verläßlich. Die Klinik ist oft verschleiert, auch die Bronchoskopie ergibt nicht zwangsläufig eine klare Diagnose, da interstitielle Prozesse nicht erfaßt werden können. Zur Diagnose einer Pneumonie sollten daher alle verfügbaren diagnostischen Möglichkeiten herangezogen werden [17, 18].

Schwierig ist zudem der Keimnachweis. Der Nachweis der Besiedlung des oberen Gastrointestinaltrakts (GIT), möglicherweise durch eine Streßulkusprophylaxe begünstigt, ist nicht beweisend für das Vorhandensein des gleichen Keims in der Lunge. Hier ist sicher die bronchoskopische Lavage hilfreich zur Keimbestimmung. Gelingt kein eindeutiger Keimnachweis, so muß eine kalkulierte Chemotherapie eingeleitet werden. Diese setzt sich aus empirisch wirksamen Substanzen gegen die nachgewiesenen Keime im oberen GIT und die im Pharynx, sowie auf den Wunden, isolierten Erreger zusammen.

Prognostisch bedeutsamste Indikation für die Antibiotikatherapie ist die generalisierte Infektion. Der Begriff „Sepsis" hat in den letzten Jahrzehnten eine bedeutende inhaltliche Wandlung erfahren. Wir verstehen darunter nicht länger nur die mit positiven Bakteriämien einhergehenden Allgemeininfektionen, sondern die Reaktion des Immunsystems des Wirtes auf auslösende Noxen. Diese können aus Bakterien oder deren Bestandteilen (z.B. Endotoxin oder Exotoxin) aber auch aus Bezirken avitalen oder minderperfundierten Gewebes bestehen.

Leider ist es trotz des Einsatzes immer neuer, immer potenterer Antibiotika nicht gelungen, die Letalität einer manifesten Sepsis zu senken. Dies hat mehrere Gründe:

1. Die Diagnose kam zu spät. Die Diagnose Sepsis kann sicher nicht mehr am positiven Blutkulturnachweis festgemacht werden, da selbst in exzellenten Serien die Inzidenz positiver Kulturen 50% nicht übersteigt. Bei zu später Diagnose ist abhängig vom invadierenden Keim eine Reaktionskette in Gang gesetzt, die möglicherweise schon zu irreversiblen Gewebeschäden in einem Ausmaß geführt hat, das nicht mehr durch Vernichtung der ursprünglich verantwortlichen Keime umzukehren ist [3].
2. Die Antibiotika verschlimmern durch Bakteriolyse mit der Freisetzung weiterer toxischer Metaboliten das bestehende Bild. Diese Reaktion, bei Staphylokokken bekannt und als Herxheimersche Reaktion bezeichnet, wird durchaus auch bei gramnegativen Species beobachtet und hat im eigenen Kollektiv zu Überlegungen geführt, im Experiment den Einsatz von Eicosanoid-Zyklus-Blockern vor der Antibiotikagabe zu prüfen.
3. Die Antibiotika sind nicht wirksam und können den septischen Prozeß nicht stoppen. Alternativ dazu besteht die Möglichkeit, daß ein pathogener Erreger vernichtet wird, gleichzeitig aber in seiner schädlichen Wirkung durch einen anderen, resistenten Keim ersetzt wird. Dieses Phänomen beobachtete Border bei der Analyse seiner positiven Blutkulturen. Antibiotika in diesem Kollektiv eliminierten zwar Keime aus dem Blut, senkten aber nicht die Inzidenz positiver Blutkulturen [3].
4. Die Antibiotika werden unterdosiert gegeben. Erstaunlich wenig ist über die Kinetik der Antibiotika bei Schwerverbrannten bekannt. Der Verlust von Körperflüssigkeiten über die großen Wundflächen macht eine Kinetikberechnung außerordentlich schwierig. Bestimmte Hersteller empfehlen bei solch kritisch Kranken, immer mit Rücksicht auf eventuell vorhandene Funktionsstörungen der Niere, per se höhere Dosierungen, um die Gefahr der Unterdosierung zu minimieren.

Schwieriger noch wird diese Situation wenn der Patient hämofiltriert wird. Hier liegen erst für einige Substanzen Erfahrungen mit Dosierungsrichtlinien vor.

Empfehlungen

Aus dem oben Gesagten wird die Schwierigkeit einer suffizienten antibiotischen Therapie deutlich; sei es der Zeitpunkt der Therapie, die Dosierung oder die Wahl der Präparate. Dennoch bleiben die Antibiotika natürlich unverzichtbarer Bestand-

Tabelle 9. Indikationen für Antibiotika

Prophylaxe	Therapie
Spalthauttransplantation	Pulmonale Infektion
Debridement	Systemische Infektion
	Wundinfektion?

Tabelle 10. Erregerspektrum bei Wundinfektionen

Staphylococcus aureus sp.	60–85%
Pseudomonas aeruginosa sp.	15–30%
E. coli	25–45%
Enterokokken	45–60%
Hämolys. Streptokokken	5–10%
Candida alb.	5–35%
Serratia marc.	0–5%
Acinetobacter cloac.	0–5%

Analyse verschiedener Sammelstatistiken

teil der Intensivtherapie. Langfristig entscheidend für den Erfolg ist aber die Beachtung einiger Grundprinzipien (Tabelle 9):

1. Prävention, strikte Hygiene, Physiotherapie und vor allem frühe Operation stellen die beste Infektionsprophylaxe dar. Gerade in der Verbrennungsbehandlung gilt: „Das Skalpell ist noch immer das beste Antibiotikum".
2. Keine prophylaktischen Antibiotika, es sei denn für die perioperative Prophylaxe bei der Transplantation oder beim Débridement außerordentlich schwer kontaminierter Areale.
3. Gesicherte Indikation zur Therapie unter Berücksichtigung der speziellen physiologischen Veränderungen beim Verbrennungstrauma.
4. Frühzeitige Diagnose und Therapiebeginn, um eine Perpetuierung pathologischer Reaktionsmechanismen auszuschließen.
5. Ausreichende Dosierung bei suffizientem Wirksamkeitsspektrum. Entscheidend ist nicht nur die Dosierung der Antibiotika sondern auch ev. Kombinationen, die eine höhere therapeutische Sicherheit bieten.
6. Antibiotikatherapie nach Stufenplan. Bei gesicherter Resistenzprüfung – Antibiotika der älteren Generation sofern Wirksamkeit nachgewiesen. Bei unklarer Resistenzlage oder „kalkulierter" Therapie – breit abdecken, um keine Therapieversager zu provozieren. Bei unsicherer Lage lieber „etwas höher einsteigen" [13].
7. Therapieerfolg beobachten und frühzeitig Wechsel des Präparates.
8. Wahl des Präparates auch nach Nebenwirkungen und ev. Synergismen ausrichten.
9. Dauernde Anpassung des eigenen Sortiments an das veränderte Resistenzprofil durch ständige Dokumentation.

Die Antibiotikatherapie bei Brandverletzten muß auch bei einem eingefahrenen Routinebetrieb immer wieder einer kritischen Würdigung unterzogen werden. Nur dadurch erhalten wir uns die Möglichkeit den sicher gutgemeinten Mißbrauch wirksamer Präparate zu verhindern und uns deren klinische Einsetzbarkeit längerfristig zu erhalten.

Der Faktor Wirtschaftlichkeit gebietet zunehmend, die Kostenfrage im Auge zu halten. Gerade die Aufwendungen für Antibiotika machen mit bis zu 20% einen „Löwenanteil" der Gesamttherapiekosten aus. Der sinnlose Einsatz verteuert die Behandlung weiter und führt letztlich auch für die Industrie dazu, daß vom Gesetzgeber immer größerer Preisdruck ausgeübt wird. Die Budgetierung der Abteilungen ist nur noch eine Frage der Zeit. Sparsam Haushalten ohne Einbußen therapeutischer Möglichkeiten stellt sicher eine optimale Vorbereitung auf diese Zeit dar.

Die Gefahr des breitgestreuten, unkritischen Antibiotikaeinsatzes kann nicht genügend betont werden. Der wachsende Selektionsdruck, forciert wiederum die Entwicklung immer neuer Substanzen. Die neueren Entwicklungen aber übertreffen in ihrer mikrobiologischen Wirksamkeit die älteren Präparate oft nur geringfügig, klinisch sichtbare Effekte sind minimal. Schon aus dem Selbsterhaltungstrieb, weiter über potente Substanzen verfügen zu können, sollte daher der Einsatz auf berechtigte Indikationen beschränkt werden.

Diese Überlegungen als Basis des therapeutischen Konzepts ermöglichen eine differenzierte, kostengünstige Antibiotikatherapie, die dann auch längerfristig für den Patienten dauerhaft zählbare Erfolge bringt.

Literatur

1. Achauer BM, Martinez SE (1985) Burn wound pathophysiology and care. Crit Care Clin 1:47–58
2. Beard CH, Ribeiro CD, Jones DM (1975) The bacteraemia associated with burns surgery. Br J Surg 62:638–641
3. Border JR, Hassett J, LaDuca J, Seibel R, Steinberg S, Mills B, Losi P, Border D (1987) The gut origin septic states in blunt multiple trauma (ISS=40) in the ICU. Ann Surg 206:427–448
4. Boss WK, Brand DA, Acampora D, Barese S, Frazier WH (1985) Effectiveness of prophylactic antibiotics in the outpatient treatment of burns. J Trauma 25:224–227
5. Boswick JAJ (1984) Management of serious infections of burns of the upper extremities. Burns Incl Therm Inj 11:63–64
6. Boswick JAJ (1987) Patterns of infection over the past ten years. Blood culture patterns. J Burn Care Rehabil 8:46–48
7. Brater DC, Bawdon RE, Anderson SA, Purdue GF, Hunt JL (1986): Vancomycin elimination in patients with burn injury. Clin Pharmacol Ther 39:631–634
8. Brauneis J, Schroder M, Laskawi R (1990) Esophageal caustic injury in childhood. A critical elucidation with indication for esophagoscopy. Laryngorhinootologie 69:398–400
9. Dasco CC, Luterman A, Curreri PW (1987) Systemic antibiotic treatment in burned patients. Surg Clin North Am 67:57–68
10. Demling RH (1985) Burns. N Engl J Med 313:1389–1398
11. Demling RH, Lalonde C (1989) Burn Trauma. Thieme, Stuttgart, New York, 1989
12. Desai MH, Herndon DN, Abston S (1987) Candida infection in massively burned patients. J Trauma 27:1186–1188
13. Deutsch DH, Miller SF, Finley RKJ (1990) The use of intestinal antibiotics to delay or prevent infections in patients with burns. J Burn Care Rehabil 11:436–442
14. Dodd D, Stutman HR (1991) Current issues in burn wound infections. Adv Pediatr Infect Dis 6:137–162
15. Germann G. Nosokomiale Wundinfektionen. In: Infektiol. Kolloquium (Bakterielle nosokomiale Infektionen) (1986) De Gruyter: 27–38
16. Germann G, Kuipers T, Perbix W, Spilker G (1990) Die Serodiagnostik der systemischen Pilzinfektion beim Schwerverbrannten. 8. Tagung DAV, Mürren 3.–6. 1. 1990

17. Goodwin CW (1984) Current burn treatment. Adv Surg 18:145–176
18. Guilbaud J, Dhennin C, Carsin H (1984) Role of Pseudomonas aeruginosa in infection in burn patients. Presse Med 13:825–829
19. Haburchak DR, Pruitt BAJ (1978) Use of systemic antibiotics in the burned patient. Surg Clin North Am 58:1119–1132
20. Herndon DN, Langner F, Thompson P, Linares HA, Stein M, Traber DL (1987) Pulmonary injury in burned patients. Surg Clin North Am 67:31–46
21. Herndon DN, Thompson PB, Traber DL (1985) Pulmonary injury in burned patients. Crit Care Clin 1:79–96
22. Hummel RP (ed) Clinical Burn Therapy. John Wright PSG, Boston Bristol London 1982
23. Jarrett F, Balish E, Moylan JA, Ellerbe S (1978) Clinical experience with prophylactic antibiotic bowel suppression in burn patients. Surgery 83:523–527
24. Krizek TJ, Koss N, Robson MC (1975) The current use of prophylactic antibiotics in plastic and reconstructive surgery. Plast Reconstr Surg 55:21–32
25. Loebl EC, Marvin JA, Heck EL, Curreri PW, Baxter CR (1974) The method of quantitative burn-wound biopsy cultures and its routine use in the care of the burned patient. Am J Clin Pathol 61:20–24
26. Lowbury EJ, Lilly HA, Kidson A, Ayliffe GA, Jones RJ (1969) Sensitivity of Pseudomonas aeruginosa to antibiotics: emergence of strains highly resistant to carbenicillin. Lancet 2:448–452
27. McManus WF, Mason ADJ, Pruitt BAJ (1980) Subeschar antibiotic infusion in the treatment of burn wound infection. J Trauma 20:1021–1023
28. MacMillan BG (1981) The control of the burn wound. Intens Care Med 7:63–69
29. Monafo WW (1979) Supportive therapy in burn care. An overview of infection control. J Trauma 19:879–880
30. Müller FE (1980) Chemotherapie und Chemoprophylaxe der Infektionen Brandverletzter. Unfallheilkunde 83:1–5
31. Opferkuch W, Lehners T (1991) Mikrobiologische Diagnostik und antimikrobielle Chemotherapie. Hippokrates, Stuttgart
32. Petersen SR, Umphred E, Warden GD (1982) The incidence of bacteremia following burn wound excision. J Trauma 22:274–279
33. Settle JA (1985) Infection in burns. J Hosp Infect 6 Suppl B:19–29
34. Simon C, Stille W (1985) Antibiotika-Therapie in Klinik und Praxis. Schattauer, Stuttgart
35. Stoutenbeek CP, van Saene HKF, Miranad DR, Zandstra DF, Binnendijk B (1984) The effect of selective decontamination of the digestive tract on colonization and infection rate in multiple trauma patients. Intens Care. Med 10:185–192
36. Talley JH (1991): Fluoroquinolones. New miracle drugs? Postgrad Med 89:101–103, 106
37. van Saeen HKF, Thülig B, Hartenauer U (1989) Antibiotikatherapie in der Intensivmedizin. In: Lawin P (Hrsg) Praxis der Intensivbehandlung. Thieme Verlag, Stuttgart New York
38. Walton MA, Carino E, Herndon DN, Heggers JP (1991) The efficacy of Polysporin First Aid Antibiotic Spray (polymyxin B sulfate and bacitracin zinc) against clinical burn wound isolates. J Burn Care Rehabil 12:116–119
39. Waymack JP (1990) Antibiotics and the postburn hypermetabolic response. J Trauma 30:S30–S33
40. Zaer F, Deodhar L (1989) Nosocomial infections due to Acinetobacter calcoaceticus. J Postgrad Med 35:14–16
41. Zellner PR, Metzger E (1977) Asepsis and antisepsis in the treatment of burn patients Infection. 5:36–45

Anschrift des Verfassers:
Priv. Doz. Dr. G. Germann
BG Unfallklinik Ludwigshafen
Abt. für Verbrennungen, Plastische- und Handchirurgie
Ludwig-Guttmann-Str. 13
D-67071 Ludwigshafen-Oggersheim

Human monoclonal antibodies for therapy of *Pseudomonas* infections

D. Rohm

Biotest Pharma GmbH, Dreieich

In spite of the use of antibiotics *Pseudomonas aeruginosa* still causes severe problems. Pollack and Young [13] and Cross et al. [2] could show that patients with high antibody titers to endotoxin have a better prognosis than patients with low or no titer. Pennington et al. [11] reported in 1986 on the efficacy of intravenous immunoglobulin treatment of experimental *Pseudomonas aeruginosa* pneumonia. Therefore, immunoglobulins derived from human plasma are used as a supportive therapy to prevent systemic *Pseudomonas* infections resulting in pneumonia and septicaemia.

For several years now, scientists have tried to establish cell lines which produce monoclonal antibodies in order to provide monoclonal antibody preparations with high titers to *Pseudomonas aeruginosa*.

What is the advantage of a monoclonal preparation compared to a plasma derived product?

1) Immunoglobulins made from a plasma pool can only provide a statistically mean value of titers to different antigens, based on the immunoglobulin pattern of the individual donors. A high specific titer in monoclonal preparations can be established by selecting antibodies with high affinity and by increasing the amount in the preparation.
2) Production of specific high titered plasma-derived immunoglobulins requires a cost intensive screening program. A monoclonal preparation from cell lines guarantees easier reproducible specificity and is cheaper to produce.
3) In general, immunoglobulins can be regarded as safe products: monoclonals may guarantee higher safety as they can be fermented, in most cases, serumfree, and intensive purification procedures lead to high virus decontamination.
4) A subclass of the monoclonals can be chosen selectively to achieve the best biological effector function.

Disadvantage

High selective reactivity of the monoclonals. Therefore a cocktail of different monoclonal antibodies has to be generated very carefully in order to give broad reactivity to the different strains of *Pseudomonas aeruginosa*.

Monoclonal antibody-producing cell lines can be made by:

1) Immortalization of human peripheral blood lymphocytes (PBLs) by EBV transformation.

2) Fusion of human PBLs with a murine myeloma or heterohybridoma cells.
3) Isolation of antibody producing genes from PBLs and transfer to producer lines (genetic engineering).

Antibody-producing cell lines are propagated in Hollow Fiber Modules or Fermenters in mass culture. The bulk harvests undergo several chromatographic steps, including virus decontamination steps, resulting in highly purified and virus safe products. These procedures are strictly regulated by guidelines of the European Community on monoclonals and biotechnology. The production must also follow Good Manufacturing Practice. Batch release is also based on the regulations of the European Pharmakopoe for Immunoglobulins from plasma (sterility, test for abnormal toxicity etc.).

Virulence factors [8, 6] and pathogenesis [17, 14, 1] of *Pseudomonas aeruginosa* have been investigated intensively during the last two decades.

Monoclonals were mainly made against three factors: Endotoxins, Flagella, Exotoxin A.

Pier et al. [12] and Suzuki et al. [16] investigated monoclonal antibodies to LPS-O side-chain of subclass G, M, and A. All three subclasses elicited in vitro opsonophagocytic killing activity in conjunction with complement in the presence of human polymorphonuclear cells (PMN) and peripheral blood monocytes (PBM). All three subclasses showed good protective activity in normal and neutropenic mice. Efficacy of LPS-O-side chain IgM monoclonals in opsonophagocytic activity tests and in protection of murine burn-wound sepsis was confirmed by Lang et al. [5]. Neely et al. [7] demonstrated efficacy of such antibodies when given pre-sepsis and post-sepsis (not later than 18 h after challenge) in this model.

Montie et al. [5] showed that motile *Pseudomonas aeruginosa* strains were much more lethal than others in burned mouse models. Holder et al. [3] demonstrated that mice immunized with flagella antigen are protected against motile *Pseudomonas* strains in this model.

Ochi et al. [9] revealed high efficacy of IgM monoclonal antibody to flagella when administered 1 h after challenge in a burned mouse model.

Kuriyama et al. [4] produced a human IgG 2 monoclonal antibody with high neutralizing in vitro and in vivo activity to Exotoxin A. The same was found by Ohtsuka et al. [10] with human IgG 3 monoclonal antibody. *These results indicate that monoclonal antibodies are highly effective in animal models and may also be of benefit in humans in severe clinical situations.*

Clinical situation:

Recently, Louis Saravolatz et al. [15] from the Henry Ford Hospital in Detroit, Michigan, reported on the first clinical trial with *Pseudomonas* monoclonal antibodies.

They combined five human IgM monoclonals directed to LPS Fischer type 1, 2, 3/7, 4 and 6, and one monoclonal of human IgG 1 type with neutralizing capacity of *Pseudomonas aeruginosa* Exotoxin A into a polyvalent preparation.

Safety, pharmaco-kinetics, and functional activity in 12 non-infected patients and eight patients with *Pseudomonas aeruginosa* bacteremia or pneumonia (or both) have been studied.

1) The preparation was well tolerated over a dose range of 0.75–3.0 mg/Kg IgM protein.
2) After a single infusion of 3.0 mg/Kg IgM, serum antibody titers were boosted into a therapeutic range (>4 µg/ml on the basis of experimental studies in animal models).
3) Serum half-lives range from 34 to 99 h.
4) Opsonophagocytic activity in serum rose more than 1 $\log_{10}$ for all but one antibody.
5) In no patient an immunologic response against the MAB preparation was detected.

At the moment we are also currently testing in a pilot study a Pseudomonas antibody cocktail of three monoclonal IgM directed against the LPS-O side chain, the outer core region of LPS, and flagella b-type.

Preclinical information:
1) The cocktail reacts with 78% of hospital isolates of *Pseudomonas*.
2) The cocktail showed
   – high in vitro activity in opsonophagocytic tests
   – protective activity in burned mice models
   – anti infectious activity in leukopenic and normal mice; the cocktail provided synergistic effects in survival rate of mice in combination with carbapenems (IPM/CS) or aminoglycosides (tobramycin, gentamicin)
   – protective activity in combination with antibiotics in intranasal infection in mice and intratracheal infection in rats.
3) Half-life in rats was examined to be 34.7 to 39.3 h. Significant amounts of i.v. administered monoclonals could be found in bronchoalveolar lavage fluid in rat lung inflamed with Exotoxin A1–2 h after treatment, but not in normal lungs.
4) Acute toxicity was studied in rats with 30 times the human dose. No adverse symptom was noticed.
5) No drop in blood pressure was observed in a rat circulatory model.
6) Cross-reactivity studies in human tissues showed no evidence of cross reactivity.
7) No viruses were detected in the fermenter and purified product. Murine and human DNA was below the detection limit.
8) Unspecific complement binding reaction is zero; no adverse signs occurred in abnormal toxicity studies.

Clinical information:
1) A few patients with severe pneumonia or burns have been treated.
2) The preparation was well tolerated after i.v. application of 20 mg per dose on 3 consecutive days dosing. No side-effects, drop of blood pressure or increase of IgE levels were detected.
3) One dose boosts serum titers into the therapeutic range (0.1 µg/ml for one, 1 µg/ml for the two other MABs). Application of three doses resulted in sufficient titers over several days.

The results of both studies indicate, that
1) monoclonal preparations are well tolerable,
2) therapeutic levels can be reached and kept for several days.

Clinical efficacy has still to be shown by ongoing studies.

References

1. Bjornson AB, Michael JG (1972) Contribution of humoral and cellular factors to the resistance to experimental infection by Pseudomonas aeruginosa in mice. II: opsonic, agglutinative, and protective capacities of immunoglobulin G anti-Pseudomonas antibodies. Infection and Immunity 5:775–782
2. Cross AS, Sadoff JC, Iglewski BH, Sokol PA (1980) Evidence for the role of toxin A in the pathogenesis of infection with Pseudomonas aeruginosa in humans. J Infect Dis 142:538–546
3. Holder A, Wheeler R, Montie TC (1982) Flagellar preparations from Pseudomonas aeruginosa: animal protection studies. Infect Immunity 35:276–280
4. Kuriyama M, Ichimori Y, Iwasa S, Trukamoto K (1990) A human-human hybridoma secreting anti-Pseudomonas aeruginosa Exotoxin A monoclonal antibody with highly potent neutralizing activity. Cytotechnology 3:31–37
5. Lang AB, Fürer E, Larrick JW, Cryz SJ (1989) Isolation and characterization of a human monoclonal antibody that recognizes epitopes shared by Pseudomonas aeruginosa immunotype 1, 3, 4 and 6 lipopolysaccharides. Infection and Immunity, 3851–3855
6. Montie TC, Doyle-Huntzinger D, Craven RC, Holder IA (1982) Loss of virulence associated with absence of flagellum in an isogenic mutant of Pseudomonas aeruginosa in the burned-mouse model. Infect Immunity 38:1296–1298
7. Neely AN, Holder IA, Larrick JW, Chong KT (1990) Comparison of preversus post-sepsis treatment with polyclonal immunoglobulin versus O serotype specific monoclonal antibody in burned Pseudomonas aeruginosa infected mice. Serodiagnosis and Immunotherapy in Infectious Disease 4:221–230
8. Nicas TI, Iglewski BH (1985) The contribution of exoproducts to virulence of Pseudomonas aeruginosa. Canadian Journal of Microbiology, 31:387–392
9. Ochi H, Ohtsuka H, Yokota SI, Uezumi I, Terashima M, Irie K, Noguchi H (1991) Inhibitory activity on bacterial motility and in vivo protective activity of human monoclonal antibodies against Flagella of Pseudomonas aeruginosa. Infect Immun 59 (2):550–554
10. Ohtsuka H, Higuchi A, Nomura N, Horigome K, Kohzuki T, Nakamori Y, Noguchi H (1992) The carboxyl terminal amino acid residues of Pseudomonas aeruginosa Exotoxin A involved in cell toxicity and pathogenesis, characterized by a neutralizing human monoclonal antibody. Biochemical and Biophysical Research Communications Vol. 180, No. 3:1498–1504
11. Pennington JE, Pier GB, Small GJ (1986 Efficacy of intravenous immune globulin for treatment of experimental pseudomonas aeruginosa pneumonia. J of Critical Care, Vol. 1, No. 1 (March), 4–10.
12. Pier GB, Thomas D, Small G, Siadak A, Zweerink H (1989) In vitro and in vivo activity of polyclonal and monoclonal human immunoglobulins G, M and A against Pseudomonas aeruginosa lipopolysaccharide. Infection and Immunity 174–179
13. Pollack M, Young LS (1979) Protective activity of antibodies to exotoxin A and lipopolysaccharide at the onset of Pseudomonas aeruginosa septicemia in man. J Clin Invest 63:276–286
14. Reynolds HY, Kazmierowski JA, Newball HH (1975) Specificity of opsonic antibodies to enhance phagocytosis of Pseudomonas aeruginosa by human alveolar macrophages. J Clin Invest 56:376–385
15. Saravolatz L, Markowitz N, Collins MS, Bogdanoff D, Pennington JE (1991) Safety, Pharmacokinetics, and Functional Activity of Human Anti-Pseudomonas aeruginosa Monoclonal Antibodies in Septic and Nonseptic Patients. J Infect Dis 164:803–806
16. Suzuki H, Okubo Y, Moriyama M, Sasaki M, Matsumoto Y, Hozumi T (1987) Human monoclonal antibodies to Pseudomonas aeruginosa produced by EBV-transformed cells. Microbiol. Immunol. Vol. 31 (10): 959–966
17. Young LS (1972) Human immunity to Pseudomonas aeruginosa: II: relationsship between heat-stable opsonins and type-specific lipopolysaccharides. J Infect Dis 126:277–287

Author's address:
Dr. D. Rohm
BIOTEST Pharma Entwicklung
Postfach 401108
D-63303 Dreieich

Measurement of sepsis in the burn patient*

A. M. Munster, M. Smith-Meek, D. Zhou, C. Dickerson and R. A. Winchurch

Baltimore Regional Burn Center; Department of Surgery, Johns Hopkins University, Baltimore, Maryland, USA

Septicemia is the 13th leading cause of death in the United States and its annual cost is estimated between $5–10 billion [2]. Much attention has been focused on gram-negative septicemia and on endotoxemia in surgical patients over recent years and a variety of therapeutic modalities have been attempted [1, 6, 8, 13]. Polymyxin B, a cationic polypeptide with anti-endotoxin effects has been used as an anti-endotoxin agent for a considerable amount of time [9] and was recently confirmed to be of value as an extracorporeal fiber filter [3] that offered improved survival in thermally injured mice [5].

More recently, the therapy of gram-negative endotoxemia and of endotoxin shock has been approached by the use of human antiserum to a mutant J5 strain of E. Coli [1, 18]. The same J5 mutant cells have been used to immunize murine splenocytes to provide IgM anti-lipid A antibody (E5) which produces a significant reduction in 30-day mortality in patients with suspected gram-negative sepsis [7]. Success has also been reported with HA1A, a human IgM antibody which is specific for lipid A, also derived from J5 immunization. In this latter series, patients with gram-negative sepsis benefitted even in the presence of septic shock [9].

These efforts have all been directed at the prevention or treatment of impending, suspected or existent gram negative sepsis. However, there is considerable evidence in the literature, particularly in burn patients, that endotoxemia exists in burned plasma early after the injury, and that its height is related to burn size [17]. It is likely that this early endotoxemia in patients with major burns is correlated with increased intestinal permeability, recently demonstrated by measurement of the lactulose mannitol excretion ratio, which could be correlated with clinical infection within the first two postburn weeks [10]. Several years ago, we began the prospective prophylaxis of patients with major burns with the administration of very small doses of polymyxin [4] and reported an improvement in immunological parameters following the therapy. The current series represents a prospective randomized study of 64 patients who received intravenous polymyxin B for the first 2 weeks after admission for major burns. The results were monitored by a sepsis scale developed by us for this purpose [11], by the chromogenic quantitative limulus lysate assay of plasma samples, and by measurements of the proinflammatory cytokine interleukin-6 (IL-6).

---

* Supported by a grant from the Metro Fire Fighters Burn Center Fund, Inc. and the Baltimore Regional Burn Center Foundation, Inc.

Materials and Methods

Patients

Patients over 18 years of age admitted to the Baltimore Regional Burn Center were enrolled following informed consent, and were randomized to a polymyxin or a control group. Polymyxin patients began therapy within 24 h of admission with intravenous polymyxin B 1500 µ/kilo/day which was increased by day 7 to 5000 µ and then decreased back to 1500 µ on day 14, at which time therapy was discontinued. No other therapeutic maneuvers normally carried out in the burn patient population were altered. Specifically, the patients were aggressively operated on with excisional surgery and early wound closure; antibiotic therapy, both topical and systemic, was carried out as clinically indicated, and ordinary monitoring and resuscitation measures were employed.

Chromogenic Limulus Lysate Assay

Plasma endotoxin was measured by the chromogenic limulus lysate assay. In principle, the assay depends on activation of a proenzyme in the limulus lysate of endotoxins. The activated enzyme catalyzes the hydrolysis of p-nitroaniline (pNA) from the colorless substrate acetylcholine-isoleucine-glutamicacid-arginine-p-nitroaniline (Ac-Ile-Glu-Arg-pNA). The release of pNA is directly proportional to the concentration of endotoxin and is quantitated by absorbance at 405 nm. With the use of well-defined endotoxin standards, a curve is generated from which the concentration of endotoxin in unknown samples can be determined.

For the assay, 100 µl samples are dispensed into pyrogen-free borosilicate tubes and brought to a temperature of 37 °C. One hundred microliters of freshly reconstituted limulus lysate was added, and the incubation was then continued for 10 min. Substrate (200 µl) is added, and the incubation was continued for an additional 3 min. The reaction was stopped by the addition of 200 µl 50 % acetic acid. The absorbance of standards and samples was measured at 405 nm. Background absorbance of reagent blanks and diluted plasma were subtracted, and the endotoxin concentration was computed from a linear equation derived from measured absorbencies of standards that ranged from 0.1 to 1.0 U/ml endotoxin. The levels of endotoxin in the samples were corrected for dilution, and the endotoxic concentration was expressed as units per milliliter.

The normal range in our laboratory was determined to be 0 to 0.1 units, which is equivalent to 0 to 10 pg/ml. Values above that are reported as "positive".

The Baltimore Sepsis Scale

There are 13 parameters of selected organ functions measured on a variable point scale. An example of how the scoring system operates is as follows: creatinine level, for each 2 mg above 2 mg is assigned a score of one point. If the patient is receiving renal dialysis, the maximum score of five points is allotted for that day. The most deviant score for the day is used to construct the score. Since no maximum points are assigned to most of the parameters that are measured, it would be theoretically possible to accumulate several hundred points a day. In practice, however, the highest score that was obtained by any patient at any time was 50.

Of the 67 patients who were employed in the polymyxin study, adequate data were available for analysis of the sepsis score in 64, and they form the basis of this report.

In the first 28 patients, the sepsis scale was not yet completely developed; therefore, to this group of patients, the sepsis scale was measured retrospectively via the hospital chart. The group of patients beginning with number 29 was studied with the sepsis scale prospectively.

IL-6 assay

The levels of IL-6 were determined with the B9 assay. For the assay, 10 units of standard IL-6 (Endogen Laboratories, Boston, Mass.) or serum samples were serially diluted in $\log_2$ increments in microtiter plates in duplicate. Log-phase B9 cells were added at a final concentration of 1×10^4 in 50 µl volumes and the plates were incubated for 3 days at 37 °C. Tritiated thymidine was added for the final 4 h of incubation, and proliferation was determined by scintillation counts.

Statistical analysis

The analysis of death or survival day-by-day, sepsis score difference between polymyxin and control patients day-by-day, and sepsis score of survivors vs. deaths day-by-day was performed by Student's *t*-test, as was the comparison of overall mean IL-6, sepsis score and endotoxin concentration. Mortality was analyzed by chi-square.

Results

Sixty-four patients completed the trial with 551 samples analyzed. A summary of the results is shown in Table 1. As can be seen, the burn size and age are well matched in the two groups. The total mortality rate with 64 patients was 12 deaths, or 18 %, but there was no difference in the mortality between polymyxin treated and control patients. There is a dramatic reduction in the mean endotoxin concentration from

Table 1. Control vs. polymyxin

	Control ($n=28$)	PB ($n=36$)	p
Burn size (%)	43.6 ± 3.4	42.4 ± 2.9	NS
Age	39.0 ± 3.2	35.4 ± 2.2	NS
Mortality	5/28	7/36	NS
Mean endotoxin (picograms/ml)	54 ± 10	21 ± 5	<0.001
Mean IL-6 (units)	1241 ± 531	380 ± 83	$<0.1 \; >0.05$
Mean sepsis score	12.5 ± 0.53	9.7 ± 0.50	<0.001

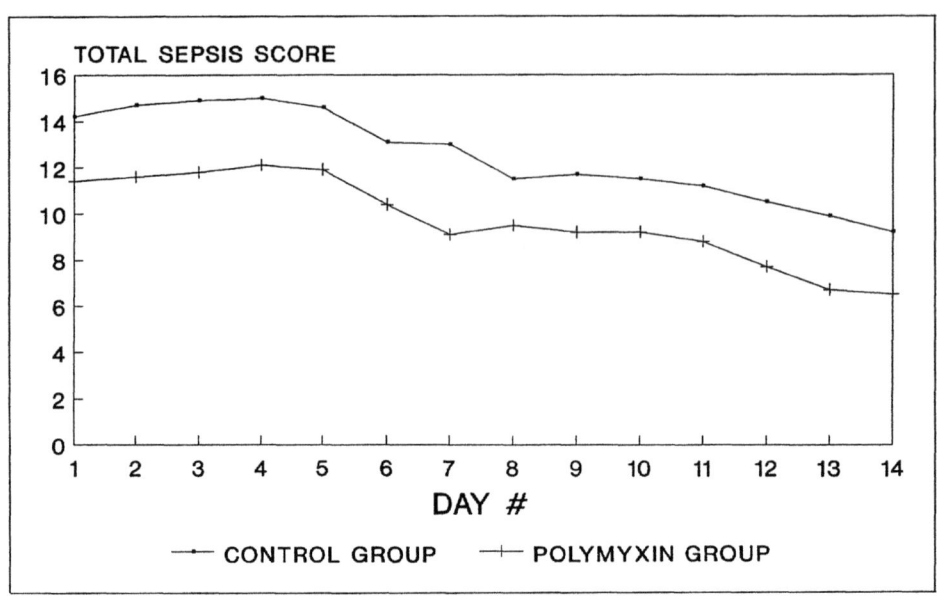

Fig. 1. Average total sepsis score for control group vs. polymyxin group

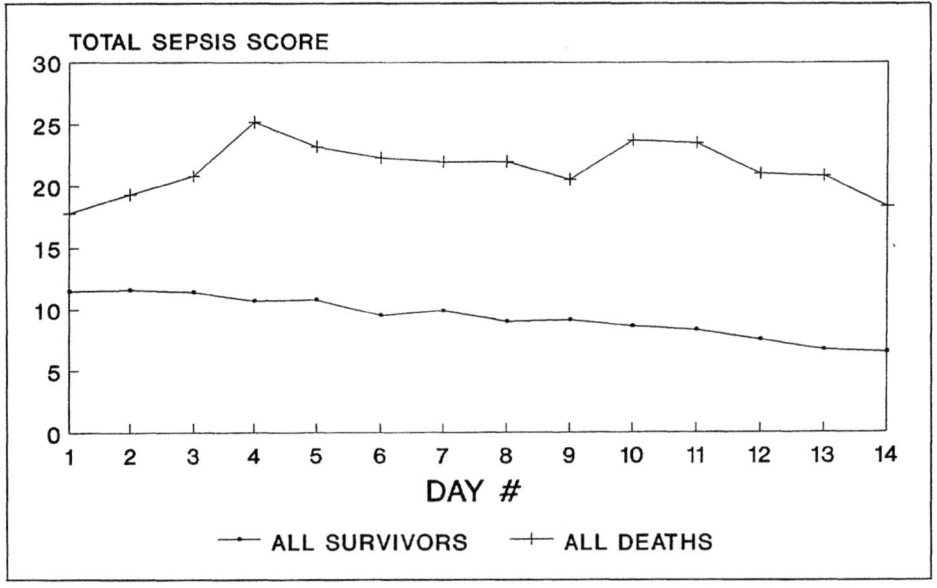

Fig. 2. Average total sepsis score for all survivors vs. all deaths

54 picograms/ml in the control group to 21 picograms/ml in the polymyxin group, which is highly statistically significant. Matching this reduction is a somewhat less dramatic, but still statistically significant reduction in the sepsis score from 12.5 to 9.7. Perhaps the most dramatic reduction following is that in IL-6 levels from 1.241 to 380 units which, however, just misses statistical significance at the p 0.05 level because of the wide standard deviation among the controls.

The above data show *means* over the 14-day study period. When analyzed on the basis of day-by-day comparison, the results become even more interesting and are shown in the next two figures. The total sepsis score for the two groups is shown in Fig. 1. It can be seen that the effect of polymyxin on the reduction of the sepsis score is immediate within the first 24 h and is maintained through the 14-day study period. The sepsis score for deaths versus survivors is shown in Fig. 2. In this figure it may be observed that the patients who will survive begin at a lower level of sepsis score and steadily lower the sepsis score at the end of day 14 from an average entry level of 11.46 and an average end level of 6.48 for survivors versus an entry point of 17.75 for deaths versus an end point of 18.3 for deaths. In other words, untreated patients maintain an up-and-down septic course for the first 2 weeks with not much difference between the beginning and the end point, whereas the polymyxin patients show a progressive improvement. When analyzed day-by-day, these data are significant or highly significant on every one of the 14 days analyzed.

The IL-6 and endotoxin data cannot be shown in this format because of irregularities and missed days in the sampling procedure and occasional technical problems that led to loss of data on certain days.

Discussion

The correlation between the resuscitation, burns, and endotoxemia is not yet clear. Recent data show that endotoxemia itself promotes translocation, as does the burn injury and resuscitation following the burn injury, but that in the absence of additional insults translocated bacteria are cleared by 96 h postburn [15]. It is also known that endotoxin induces IL-6 messenger RNA expression in multiple organs following experimental injection, peaking at 1 to 2 h after injection [16]. Tumor necrosis factor and IL-1 also induce IL-6 expression; IL-6 in turn inhibits TNF and IL-1 mRNA expression and this system resembles a feedback loop. The expression and eventual secretion of IL-6 from many sites is probably connected with the induction of a large family of lipopolysaccharide binding proteins involved in responses to gram-negative sepsis which are produced in the hepatocyte, the neutrophil, the macrophage, and in murine B-cells [14]. These lipopolysaccharide binding proteins are responsible at least in part for host effects against gram-negative sepsis, which is teleologically a very ancient reaction. In man, although endotoxemia of limited degree seems useful because of the induction of acute phase response mobilizing cytokine responses, when these responses are overwhelmed, clinical septic shock and death ensues. If, therefore, translocational endotoxemia early after injury is possibly responsible for inducing a vicious cycle of further translocation and multiple organ failure, then the interruption of this vicious cycle early in the course after injury should be at least theoretically useful.

Our results with the elevation of IL-6 corresponding to increasing sepsis score and thereby the clinical development of sepsis is in line with previous reports which correlate the severity of illness in burn patients with the height of IL-6 level [12, 20]. Our inability to demonstrate any reduction in mortality is disappointing, but needs to be viewed in the context of *overall* mortality and sometimes, several months after the cessation of polymyxin treatment, as opposed to early preventive measures by the polymyxin against translocational endotoxemia only. At no point did we attempt to actually treat a patient with polymyxin or any other agent and, therefore, the potential utility of polymyxin in the same setting as the earlier quoted reports on HA1A and E5 is unknown. Since the threat of death from sepsis to burn patients is practically ubiquitous until the time of discharge, be it from pulmonary complications, from late occurring intravenous line sepsis, or from late sequelae of burn-wound sepsis, it would be unreasonable to expect that control of early translocational endotoxemia would prevent late mortality. To accomplish that, therapeutic approaches will need to be employed with polymyxin-B or other similar agents.

Summary

In a prospective randomized study of 64 patients with major burns, therapy for prophylaxis of endotoxemia was performed with the use of intravenous polymyxin B in small doses. The polymyxin and control groups were well matched for age, burn size, and incidence of inhalation injury. There was no reduction in mortality in the polymyxin group. There was a highly significant reduction of the mean endotoxin concentration in the polymyxin group and in the mean sepsis score of the polymyxin group; there was an impressive reduction in the IL-6 level of the polymyxin group, however, because of the wide standard deviation that difference did not reach statistical significance. We conclude that endotoxemia, probably as a result of intestinal translocation, is a clinically relevant phenomenon, and its control by measures aimed at lipid A neutralization is possible. It does not, alone, account for mortality and, therefore, to reduce mortality from clinical sepsis later in the course of the patient's illness, therapeutic intervention at those times will need to be added to anti-translocational prophylaxis.

References

1. Baumgartner JD, Glauser MP, McCutchan JA et al. (1985) Prevention of gram-negative shock and death in surgical patients by antibody to endotoxin core glycolipid. Lancet 2:59–63
2. Centers for Disease Control (1987) Increase in national hospital discharge survey rates for septicemia – U.S. 1979–1987. MMWR 39:31–34
3. Cheadle WG, Hanasawa K, Gallinaro RN, Nimmanwudipong T, Kodama M, Polk Jr. HC (1991) Endotoxin filtration and immune stimulation improve survival from gram-negative sepsis. Surgery 110:785–792
4. Chiccone TG, Munster AM, Birmingham W and Winchurch RA (1983) Successful immunomodulation in burned animals and humans with homeopathic doses of polymyxin B. JBCR 4:153
5. Crowley BM, Riordain G, Ellwanger K, Collins KH, Saporoschetz IB, Pilz MA, Mannick JA, Rodrick MD (1990) Antiendotoxin therapy improves survival in a model of thermal injury and sepsis. Surg Forum 41:72–74
6. Dunn DL, Mach PA, Condie RM, Cerra FB (1984) Anticore endotoxin F(ab')2 equine immunoglobulin fragments protect against lethal effects of gram-negative sepsis. Surgery 96:440

7. Greenman RL, Schein RMH, Martin MA et al (1991) A controlled clinical trial of E5 murine monoclonal IgM antibody to endotoxin in the treatment of gram-negative sepsis. JAMA 266:1097–1102
8. Hinshaw LB, Archer LT, Beller BK et al. (1988) Evaluation of naloxone therapy for E Coli sepsis in the baboon. Arch Surg 123:700
9. Ingoldby CJ, Gilbert AD et al. (1984) Endotoxemia in human obstructive jaundice: Effect of polymyxin B. Amer J Surg 147:766–771
10. LeVoyer T, Cioffi WG, Pratt L, Shippee R, McManus WF, Mason AD and Pruitt BA (1992) Alterations in intestinal permeability after thermal injury. Arch Surg 127:26–30
11. Meek M, Munster AM, Winchurch RA, Dickerson C (1991) The Baltimore Sepsis Scale: Measurement of sepsis in burn patients using a new scoring system. JBCR 12:564–568
12. Moran K, O'Reilly T, Thupari J, Xiao G, Winchurch RA, Karadesh D, Allo M, Munster AM (1987) Endotoxin impairs neutrophil function in burn patients. Surg Forum 38:94
13. Rubin RM, Noland J, Rosenbaum JT (1988) Monoclonal antibodies directed against endotoxin reduce endotoxin-induced vascular permeability. Clin Res 36:147a
14. Tobins PT, Mathison JC, Vleritch RJ (1988) A family of lipopolysaccharide binding proteins involved in responses to gram-negative sepsis. J Biol Chem 263:13479–13481
15. Tokyay R, Zeigler ST, Heggers JP, Loick HM, Traber DL, Herndon DN (1991) Effects of anaesthesia, surgery, fluid resuscitation, and endotoxin administration on postburn bacterial translocation. J Trauma 31:1376–1379
16. Veich TR, Guo K, Remick D, Castillo J, Yin S (1991) IL6 in RNA and serum protein expansion and the in vivo hematologic effects of IL6. J Immunol 146:2316–2323
17. Winchurch RA, Thupari JN, Munster AM (1987) Endotoxemia in burn patients: Levels of circulating endotoxins are related to burn size. Surgery 102:808
18. Ziegler EJ, McCutchan JA, Fierer J et al. (1982) Treatment of gram-negative bacteremia and shock with human antiserum to a resistant Escherichia Coli. N Eng J Med 307:1225–1230
19. Ziegler EJ, Fisher CJ, Spring CL et al. (1991) Treatment of gram-negative bacteremia and septic shock with a HA1A human monoclonal antibody against endotoxin. N Eng J Med 324:429–436
20. Zhou D, Munster AM, Winchurch RA (1992) Inhibitory effects of interleukin 6 on immunity: Possible implications in burn patients. Arch Surg 127:65–69

Author's address:
A.M. Munster, M.D.
F.R.C.S. (Eng & Ed) F.A.C.S.
Baltimore Regional Burn Center
4940 Eastern Avenue;
Baltimore, MD 21224, USA

Die Therapie der Sepsis

G. Germann

Abteilung für Plastische Chirurgie und Verbrennungskrankheiten BG-Universitätsklinik Bergmannsheil, Bochum

Definition – Inzidenz

„75 % of all deaths in a Burn ICU are due to sepsis". Dieser Satz von Pruitt gibt zwar im wesentlichen unsere klinische Erfahrung wieder, trägt aber hinsichtlich der Begriffsbestimmung oder der zugrunde liegenden pathophysiologischen Zusammenhänge wenig zur Verdeutlichung bei [57]. Kaum ein Begriff hat seit der Definition durch Schottmüller [74] in den letzten Jahrzehnten ähnlich viele inhaltliche Modifikationen und Wandlungen erfahren wie der Terminus „Sepsis". Die Begriffe „Sepsis", „Septikämie", „Bakteriämie" und „Septischer Schock" werden in der Literatur nahezu beliebig austauschbar benutzt. Das Spektrum der Definitionen reicht von einem lebensbedrohlichen Zustand, ausgelöst durch Bakterien, bis zu einer „general inflammatory response" des Körpers, die keine Präsenz von Bakterien erfordert [2, 10, 11, 37, 54, 57, 71, 76, 77, 83, 85, 92].

Eine Vielzahl klinischer und experimenteller Studien haben speziell in den letzten 20 Jahren eine kaum noch überschaubare Menge an Einzelaspekten untersucht. Die Analyse der klinischen Symptomatik, der Störungen der peripheren Perfusion und der Abläufe auf zellulärer Ebene haben zu einem neuen pathophysiologischen Gesamtverständnis dieses komplexen Geschehens geführt. Dabei sind viele experimentelle und klinische Befunde widersprüchlich und viele Fragen hinsichtlich des Zusammenspiels der beteiligten Faktoren, vor allem im Bereich der „zellulären Endstrecke" weiter ungeklärt.

Durch die Forschungsergebnisse der letzten 20 Jahre haben sich viele Lücken im Bild der Sepsis gefüllt. Es ist heute als sicher anzunehmen, daß eine „septic response" auf ein Trauma oder die Existenz ausgedehnter nekrotischer Areale z. B. nach Verbrennungen, auch ohne Keiminvasion das Vollbild der Sepsis bzw. des septischen Schocks erzeugen kann. Vielfach wird Sepsis heute als weitgehend uniforme, nur graduell abgestufte „septische Antwort" bzw. „generalisierte inflammatorische Reaktion" auf ein Spektrum unterschiedlicher Noxen betrachtet. Neue Definitionen der Sepsis wurden geschaffen um dem Kliniker alltagstaugliche Definitionen an die Hand zu geben. Neben die traditionellen infektiösen Zeichen traten vor allem die Zeichen einer gestörten Organperfusion bzw. Organfunktion. Der Zusammenhang zwischen septischem Zustandsbild des Patienten und einem eintretenden Organversagen fließt so in viele Definitionen der Sepsis ein [1, 2, 10, 11, 36, 54, 55, 58, 66, 76, 83, 92] (Tabelle 1).

Ungeachtet der benutzten Definition ist das septische Krankheitsbild gerade für den schwerst immunsupprimierten Verbrannten von entscheidender prognostischer Bedeutung. Trotz der zunehmenden Erkenntnisse über Pathophysiologie und Immunologie der Sepsis ist es nicht gelungen die Letalität in den letzten 10–20 Jahren entscheidend zu senken. Noch immer wird die Inzidenz der Sepsis zwischen 5–40 %,

Tabelle 1. Autoren unterschiedlicher klinischer Begriffsbestimmungen der Sepsis

- Bone
- Veterans Administration (VA)
- Sibbald
- APACHE II, III
- SIS
- MOF-Score

die der letal verlaufenden Sepsis zwischen 5–18 % angegeben [58]. Mit 50–75 % stellt die Sepsis weiterhin die Haupttodesursache bei Schwerverbrannten dar [30, 55, 103]. Das Überleben des Patienten hängt daher auch heute im wesentlichen von der Prävention bzw. Früherkennung und Beherrschung dieses Zustandes ab.

Infolge der fast „babylonisch" anmutenden Zahl von Definitionen ist es außerordentlich schwierig die Behandlungsergebnisse verschiedener Autoren in ihren Kollektiven zu vergleichen. Häufig wurden inhomogene Kollektive untersucht, in denen schon aufgrund der Eingangskriterien keine Vergleichbarkeit zwischen den einzelnen Untergruppen möglich war. Durch höchst unterschiedliche Definitionen der Kriterien des Organversagens wird zusätzlich die Beurteilung einer gestörten Organfunktion für das Kriterium Sepsis erschwert. Eine Metaanalyse der Literatur wird durch diese erheblichen Abweichungen nahezu unmöglich. Eine Konsensus Konferenz hat sich daher 1987 in den USA bemüht, Definitionen und Begriffe auf einen gemeinsamen Nenner zu bringen [2]. Allerdings dauert die Diskussion um die endgültige Fassung bis in die jüngste Vergangenheit an [10, 11, 83, 85] und ein Ende ist noch nicht absehbar.

Bevor jedoch die Therapie der Sepsis bzw. des septischen Schocks einsetzt, muß definiert sein, welches Krankheitsbild eigentlich behandelt wird. Wird eine invasive bakterielle Infektion behandelt oder therapieren wir einen physiologischen Zustand, der zur Entwicklung des Vollbildes nicht der Anwesenheit von Bakterien bedarf [37, 64]? Immerhin findet sich nur in ca 50 % der Fälle eine offensichtliche Infektionsquelle [54]. Diese Frage macht deutlich, daß am Anfang der Therapie eine eindeutige Diagnose, bzw. Definition stehen muß. Nur so sind die Inzidenz der Sepsis, Letalitätsraten und Therapieerfolge bzw. der Effekt bestimmter Medikamente in den verschiedenen Kollektiven auch nur annähernd vergleichbar [76, 79].

Die nächste Frage ist, ob die Diagnose aufgrund klinischer oder leicht zu messender Laborparameter gestellt werden soll, oder ob schwierige, nicht überall zugängliche Laboruntersuchungen durchgeführt werden müssen. Besitzen diese Laboruntersuchungen eine höhere Aussagekraft als einfache Parameter und erlauben sie eine frühere Diagnose und damit effektivere Therapie? Es stehen mittlerweile eine Vielzahl von teilweise hochspezifischen Untersuchungen zur Verfügung, mit denen nahezu alle Mediatoren und Faktoren, denen eine Rolle bei der Pathogenese der Sepsis zugeschrieben wird, gemessen werden können [39] (Tabelle 2–3).

Dazu gehören die Bestimmung der Serumspiegel von IL 2, IL 6, Endotoxin, TNF, Elastase, Hyaluronsäure, C 1 Inhibitor Komplex und der aktivierten Komplementfaktoren [7, 48] (Tabelle 4).

Als klinische Diagnosekriterien haben sich die Parameter der oben angeführten Definitionen bewährt. Auch Intensiv-Scoring Systeme die sich an physiologischen Parametern orientieren (APACHE II, SIS, MSIS, MOF-Score), erlauben eine früh-

Tabelle 2. Definition der Multicenter Studie Veterans Administration 1987

- Klinischer Verdacht auf Sepsis und 4 von 7 Kriterien
- Schüttelfrost oder Fieber (>38,9°, <35,5°)
- Tachypnoe (>28/min), Hypokapnie (<32 mmHg)
- Tachykardie (>100)
- Hypotension (<90 mmHg syst.)
- Leukozytose, -Penie (>15 000, <3 500)
- Thrombopenie (<100 000)
- Sepsisherd, chirurgischer Eingriff

Tabelle 3. Definition von Bone 1991

- Sepsis und ein oder mehrere Zeichen veminderter Organperfusion
- Mentale Veränderung
- Absacken PaO_2, Anstieg FiO_2
- Laktatanstieg
- Oligurie ($\leq$ 0,5 ml/kg/KG/h)

Tabelle 4. Sepsis. Heute meßbare spezifische Mediatoren

- Interleukin 2 (IL 2)
- Interleukin 6 (IL 6)
- TNF
- Endotoxin
- C 1 Inhibitor
- Elastase
- Hyaluronsäure
- Komplementfaktoren

zeitige Diagnosestellung, die zeitlich nicht gegenüber der Messung spezifischer Laborparameter zurückfällt. Die tägliche Erfassung dieser Scores ermöglicht darüber hinaus das Ansprechen auf unterschiedliche Therapiemaßnahmen zu dokumentieren. An validierten Kollektiven lassen sich aus diesen Bewertungssystemen auch prognostische Aussagen ableiten [17, 38, 49, 50, 61, 68, 69].

Am Beispiel eines Kollektivs schwerverbrannter Patienten (n=100, mindest. KOF=30%), die alle aufgrund der Schwere des Traumas mehr als 5 Tage beatmet werden mußten, soll die Wichtigkeit einer klaren Definition für die Aussagekraft einer Studie und die Relation zur Therapie verdeutlicht werden.

Zur Definition der Sepsis wurden die Kriterien von Bone, der VA-Studie und eine eigene „verschärfte Version" benutzt, da viele der Bone Kriterien zu „weich" erschienen. Aufgrund der Arbeiten von Carvajal, Goris und anderen wurde auf die Bestimmung von Endotoxin, IL 6 oder anderen Mediatoren verzichtet. Die Diagnosestellung erfolgte streng nach den oben erläuterten Kriterien unabhängig von der subjektiven Meinung einzelner Kollegen [17, 36, 38, 76, 79] (Tabelle 5–6).

Die Inzidenz septischer Komplikationen betrug 60%. An 1469 von 1896 Behandlungstagen erfüllten diese schwerverletzten Patienten die Kriterien der Sepsis. Die Gesamtsterblichkeit betrug 45%. Organdysfunktion oder Versagen von Organsyste-

Tabelle 5. Definition der septischen Zeichen für eine Studie zur Interaktion Sepsis und Organversagen

Thrombozyten	<75 000
Leukozyten	<5 000/>15 000
Reptilase	>25 s
Fieber	>38,5°, <35,6°
Laktat	>2,2 mg/dl
Katecholamine	>5 yg/h/kg/KG/2. Kat.
Blutkultur	positiv
Beatmung	FiO_2 >0,4
Tachykardie	>100

Tabelle 6. Definition des Organversagens für die Studie (s. Abb. 5)

Lunge	MB, FiO_2 >0,4
Niere	Kreatinin >2,0 mg/dl
Leber	Bilirubin >2 mg/dl
Kreislauf	DOP/DOB >4 yg/min/kg/KG oder 2. Katecholamin
Gerinnung	Thrombozyten <75 000
	Quick <60%
Laktat	>2,2 mg/dl

men war immer mit der Erfüllung der Definitionskriterien der Sepsis korreliert. Es ergab sich eine eindeutige sequentielle Folge des Ausfalls der Organsysteme. Die Ergebnisse zeigen, daß aufgrund der vorher bestimmten Definitionen eindeutige Aussagen zur Inzidenz der Sepsis, der zeitlichen Sequenz der organspezifischen Komplikationen und zur kausalen Korrelation zwischen Sepsis und Organversagen zu machen sind. Da die Inzidenz septischer Zeichen höher lag als zu Studienbeginn erwartet, eröffnete sich die Möglichkeit durch die konsequente tägliche Bewertung der Patienten eine drohende Sepsis früh zu erkennen und therapeutische Maßnahmen einzuleiten (Tabelle 7–8).

Organversagen – Pathophysiologie

Das Organversagen bzw. die Dysfunktion von Organen ist bei den Definitionen dieser Studie schon Bestandteil des Begriffs Sepsis. Der enge Zusammenhang zwischen der Sepsis und dem Organversagen bzw. Multiorganversagen (MOV) wird dadurch untermauert, daß alle Patienten mit Organversagen zu diesem Zeitpunkt die Kriterien der Sepsis erfüllten (s.o.). Dies bedeutet, daß die der Sepsis zugrunde liegenden pathophysiologischen Mechanismen zu diesem Zeitpunkt schon erhebliche Veränderungen der Mikrozirkulation und des zellulären Stoffwechsels in den betroffenen Organen verursacht haben [4, 16, 24, 33, 34, 36].

Um diesen circulus vitiosus nicht noch zu perpetuieren, muß als erstes die Ursache beseitigt werden. Dies bedeutet bei einem offensichtlich infizierten Fokus ein radikales Débridement. Das kann im Bereich der plastischen Chirurgie ein septischer Unterschenkel sein, bei Verbrannten sind es zumeist noch nicht exzidierte bzw. sekundär infizierte Areale („burn wound sepsis"). Ob es nun durch Keiminvasion

Tabelle 7. Inzidenz der Organbeteiligungen bei Vorliegen eines Multiorganversagens (MOV)

Lunge	74	
Kreislauf	69	
Knochenmark	57	
Leber	48	
Niere	38	$n = 100$

Tabelle 8. Inzidenz der verschiedengradigen Ausprägung des MOV

MOV 2	21 (6)	
MOV 3	23 (17)	
MOV 4	13 (10)	
MOV 5	7 (7)	
Behandlungstage	2896	
Tage mit OV	1468	$n = 100$

In Klammern Verstorbene

oder avitales verbranntes Gewebe zur Auslösung der Mediatorenketten kommt, ist von sekundärer Bedeutung. Entscheidend ist, daß die Ursache der Sepsis, soweit faßbar, eliminiert wird. Dabei muß auch eine intraoperative Keimeinschwemmung in Kauf genommen werden [26].

Dies bedeutet für unsere therapeutischen Entscheidungen, daß wir mit der Therapie der Organdysfunktion auch die Sepsis als Ganzes (und vice versa) bekämpfen. Der Kampf ähnelt dem gegen die Hydra, da es an mehreren Fronten zu einem Angriff gegen die zelluläre Integrität kommt. Einerseits besteht möglicherweise eine kontinuierliche bakterielle Invasion, zum anderen eine große Fläche avitalen, verbrannten Gewebes. Beide Faktoren können eine permanente Stimulation der Mediatorsysteme verursachen, die dann das Bild der „septic response" auslösen [84]. Zum anderen findet sich regelmäßig ein „Dominoeffekt des Organversagens", d.h. bei progredienter Dysfunktion bzw. Versagen eines Organsystems kommt es nahezu zwangsläufig zum sequentiellen Versagen anderer Systeme [4, 28, 33, 36, 38].

Ungeachtet der zugrundeliegenden Ursache kommt es in der Sepsis zu einer Aktivierung multipler körpereigener Mediatorsysteme und Abwehrmechanismen, die zu schweren Veränderungen aller Organfunktionen führen können. Schlüsselsubstanz bei bakteriell ausgelöster Sepsis ist das Endotoxin (LPA), ein Lipopolysaccharid gram-negativer Bakterien; bei nicht bakterieller Sepsis kommt es durch die untergehenden Zellen zu einer massiven Komplementaktivierung [44, 87]. An erster Stelle der körpereigenen Mediatoren sind der Tumor-Nekrose-Faktor α (TNF) und die Interleukine 1 (IL 1) und 6 (IL 6) [26, 63] aber auch die Eicosanoide (Arachidonsäurederivate) wie Prostaglandine, Thromboxan und Leukotriene sowie die Gerinnungskaskade zu nennen [65, 78]. Neueste Untersuchungen zeigen, daß eine Imbalance zwischen Thromboxan und Prostazyklin eine Rolle in der Pathogenese des MOV spielen kann [104]. Vor allem TNF löst bei Gabe als Reinsubstanz eine Vielzahl septischer Symptome aus [3, 18, 21, 27, 75]. Das Herz-Kreislauf-System ist schon früh in der Sepsis durch eine Einschränkung der kardialen Leistungsfähigkeit mitbetroffen [29, 96]. Dies hat primär noch keine Auswirkungen auf die Mikrozirkulation und die Gewebeperfusion, besitzt aber prognostischen Charakter (Tabelle 9a–b).

Tabelle 9 a, b. a) Entzündungsmediatoren (vorwiegend Monozyten und Makrophagenprodukte). **b)** Entzündungsmediatoren (vorwiegend plasmatische Faktoren)

a)

LT B4	PMN, Monozyten Makrophagen	Chemotaxis, Deg. PMN Immunregulation
LT C4	Mastzellen Makrophagen	Kontraktion, glatte Muskulatur Permeabilität
PG E2	Monozyten Makrophagen	Vasodilatation, verst. LT-Wirkung Immunsuppression
PG I2	Monozyten Makrophagen, Endothel	Vasodilatation Verbesserung Zellstoffwechsel

b)

Histamin	Mastzellen	Steigerung/Permeabilität, Kontraktion, glatte Muskulatur
Bradykinin	Kininogen	Vasodilatation, Schmerz Permeabilität
C5a	Komplementsystem	Chemotaxis, Deg. Granulozyten
C3a	Komplementsystem	Granulozyten Thrombozyten
PAF	Granulozyten, Monozyten Makrophagen	Aggregation, Aktivierung inflam. Zellen, Permeabilität

Im weiteren Verlauf kommt es aber durch die Mechanismen der Sepsis, wie im Initialtrauma der Verbrennung, zu einem kapillären Leck mit einer konsekutiven extravasalen Ödembildung, einer Steigerung der O_2-Diffusionsstrecke und einer globalen Perfusionsminderung durch die veränderte Rheologie. Kommt es zusätzlich zu einer Hypotonie (RR syst. <90 mmHg), wird der Zustand als „septischer Schock" bezeichnet. Andere Autoren definieren „septischen Schock" auch als Blutdruckabfall von mindestens 40 mmHg oder die bestehende Notwendigkeit zum Einsatz von Katecholaminen. Hypotonie über 24 h oder anhaltender Widerstandsverlust sind prognostisch ungünstig [20].

Die Gefäßendothelien werden aktiviert und anhaftende Leukozyten setzen zusätzlich direkt zytotoxische Sauerstoffradikale frei [93, 94]. Fast alle Komponenten des Sauerstofftransports sind eingeschränkt, die Verteilung in den Geweben und die Extraktion ist reduziert. Dazu tritt ein oft massiver Abfall des peripheren Widerstands (TPR) durch Öffnung arterio-venöser Shunts. Die pathologischen Veränderungen ergeben das klinische Bild der hyperdynamen Schockphase. Durch die verschlechterte Gewebeoxygenierung machen sich erste klinisch faßbare Organfunktionseinschränkungen wie auffälliges Verhalten oder Nachlassen der Ausscheidung bemerkbar. Die Körpertemperatur verliert ihre Regulationsmechanismen und der Patient wird entweder fiebrig oder hypotherm. Viele der physiologischen Veränderungen sind das Resultat der Freisetzung körpereigener Substanzen, die sonst lokal begrenzt an der Eliminierung entzündlicher Prozesse oder an normalen reparativen Vorgängen beteiligt sind. Offensichtlich entwickeln diese Prozesse bei Übergreifen auf die systemische Ebene im Gegensatz zum lokalen Geschehen eine bedeutende destruktive Potenz.

Alle Abwehrfunktionen des Immunsystems sind eingeschränkt, was sich in einer Zunahme der T-Suppressor Zellen und einer Abnahme der B-Lymphozyten und deren Proliferation zeigt. Auch die Expression wichtiger Rezeptoren und die Synthese von Zytokinen ist vermindert [8, 51, 72, 73, 106].

Definiert man Schock als Mißverhältnis zwischen angebotenem und vom Gewebe benötigtem O_2, so ist die zelluläre Dysfunktion Ausdruck eines Schockzustandes. Wichtigstes Therapieprinzip ist daher die Restitution der Zirkulation, vor allem der Mikrozirkulation und damit der Verbesserung der Gewebeoxygenierung und die Anhebung des O_2-Verbrauchs in der Peripherie, sei es durch Erhöhung der Extraktion oder Steigerung des Sauerstoffangebots (DO^2 = Oxygen Delivery) [14, 40, 42, 70, 98].

Viele der therapeutischen Ziele können schon durch ausreichende Volumengabe, die sog. „volume challenge" erreicht werden. Das intravasale Volumen wird vermehrt, die Tachykardie gesenkt und als Ergebnis der gesteigerten Auswurfleistung (Cardiac output = CO) auch die Perfusion verbessert. Der Körper versucht durch ein „capillary recruitment" die Zahl der synchron perfundierten Kapillaren zu steigern. Die Vergrößerung des Plasmavolumens kann in der Peripherie durch Erhöhung der Durchflußmenge die Aggregation von Granulozyten auflösen, die Bildung weiterer Mikrothromben verhindern, die Maldistribution des Flow korrigieren und damit die energetische Situation der Endstrombahn verbessern. Gelingt dies, so wird sich der Verlust der Mikroangiodynamik normalisieren und das Geschehen mehr in Richtung reparativer Prozesse gelenkt.

Gelingt dies nicht, so kann es im weiteren Verlauf zu einer zunehmenden Dekompensation des Stoffwechsels mit Substitution der Energiegewinnung durch anaerobe Glykolyse, einer energetischen Mangelsituation und einem progredienten Zelluntergang kommen. Die peripheren Gewebe verlieren ihre Fähigkeit zur vermehrten Sauerstoffextraktion und werden in ihrer Versorgung vom Sauerstoffangebot abhängig („oxygen supply dependency" = OSD). Es stellt sich eine periphere Sauerstoffschuld, d. h. eine Differenz zwischen kalkuliertem O_2-Verbrauch und tatsächlicher Extraktion ein. Gerade im Mesenterialbereich kann dies durch eine Steigerung der intestinalen Permeabilität zu einer vermehrten Translokation führen [32]. Je höher die angehäufte O_2-Schuld, desto schlechter die Prognose des Patienten. Der kritische O_2-Wert, d. h. der Wert bei dem eine erhöhte Sauerstoffextraktion nicht ausreicht die Sauerstoffaufnahme zu erhalten, steigt in der Sepsis von ca 8–10 ml/kg/min bis auf 21 ml/kg/min an. Dieses Phänomen wird als „oxygen supply dependency" bezeichnet und besitzt prognostischen Wert. Überlebende Patienten können ihre Sauerstoffextraktion steigern, versterbende Patienten bleiben vom Angebot abhängig. Hauptursache für die verminderte Extraktion sind Verlust der Kapillarreserve, Endothelschädigung, Mikroembolisation und zelluläre Utilisationsstörung [15, 59, 84]. Bei Irrversibilität führt dies zum klinischen Bild des Multiorganversagens [5].

Tabelle 10. Stufentherapie der Sepsis

**	→ Volumen (Antibiotika, Operation)	
Normalisierung		keine Besserung
		mehr Volumen (FFP)
**	MAK	Katecholamine
	IG	Beatmung
	NOSAC	symptomatisch
	O₂ Scavenger	

Therapie

Die primären Therapieziele müssen daher sein:

- Hebung das Cardiac output,
- Hebung des TPR,
- Normalisierung der Frequenz,
- Steigerung der Gewebedurchblutung,
- Verkleinerung der A-V Differenz,
- Senkung des kritischen DO2,
- Vermeidung einer OSD.

Zirkulation

Sehr häufig genügt die Volumengabe nicht. Dies vor allem dann, wenn das Herz des Patienten durch die Sepsis per se oder durch vorbestehende Funktionsstörungen in seiner Kontraktilitätskraft eingeschränkt ist. Gerade die kardiale Leistungsfähigkeit ist früher eingeschränkt als häufig angenommen wird [67]. Verschiedene Mediatoren wirken direkt auf Enzymsysteme der kardialen Energiegewinnung und damit auf Kontraktilität und Reizleitungssystem. Die Existenz eines sog. „myocardial depressan factor" (MDF) wird diskutiert, dieser ist aber möglicherweise eine Mischung verschiedener kleinmolekularer Peptide und ähnelt in Fragmenten dem TNF [29, 43, 62, 96].

In der Lunge kommt es zu einem erhöhten Rechts-Links Shunt Volumen, der pulmonale Widerstand ist oft erhöht und das Herz hat eine erhöhte Vorlast zu bewältigen [60]. Die „Steifigkeit" des Herzens nimmt zu, d. h. die Compliance sinkt und die Auswurfleistung nimmt ab. Dies ist aber häufig auch ein Effekt der Katecholamine, die durch Verbesserung der Vitalparameter einen Volumenmangel kaschieren können. Dennoch ist es in vielen Situationen unumgänglich Katecholamine einzusetzen [70].

Hier hat sich vor allem nach den Untersuchungen von Shoemaker Dobutamin hervorragend bewährt. Mit seiner Wirkung sowohl auf die kardialen α-Rezeptoren als auf periphere β1 Rezeptoren ist es sowohl möglich die Kontraktilität und Pumpleistung des Herzens zu verbessern als auch eine zusätzliche periphere Vasokonstriktion zur Hebung des Blutdrucks zu verhindern. Werden größere Dosen an Dobutamin gebraucht, kommt es allerdings auch hier zu einer gewissen α-adrenergen peripheren Reaktion [80, 82]. Exogene Katecholamine können außerdem die sog. koronare Reserve aktivieren [9]. Eine Kombination mit Dopamin wird in vielen Intensivstationen oft in der Vorstellung durchgeführt, die beiden Haupteffekte der Substanzen kombinieren zu können. Dopamin wirkt in niedriger Dosierung selektiv fördernd auf die Mesenterialdurchblutung, was sich klinisch als Erhöhung des Urinvolumens ausdrückt.

Die Reaktionen auf Katecholamine sind individuell und können, gerade beim Dopamin, häufig in einer Tachykardie resultieren. Daher wird man als primäres Katecholamin Dobutamin einsetzen, möglicherweise in Kombination mit Dopamin. Bei Dobutamin werden vereinzelt nach einer Therapiedauer von 48 h Tachyphylaxie ähnliche Erscheinungen beobachtet, die eine kontinuierliche Dosiserhöhung erfordern. Indikationen für die beiden anderen, therapeutisch verfügbaren Katecholamine gibt es eigentlich nur noch für den Ausnahmefall. Hier haben aber sowohl Adrenalin als auch Noradrenalin ihren Platz.

Es kommt unter Noradrenalin zu einer massiven Konstriktion der Peripherie, was sicher die metabolische Situation der Zellen weiter verschlechtert, aber den Blutdruck in den noch durchbluteten Arealen stabilisiert. Es gelingt den totalen peripheren Widerstandverlust zu durchbrechen und die hyperdyname Kreislaufsituation hierdurch zu bessern. Adrenalin ist ebenfalls ein potenter α-adrenerger Stimulator, besitzt aber eine größere Fähigkeit der kardialen Leistungssteigerung. Auch Noradrenalin verfügt, im Gegensatz zu früheren Annahmen, durchaus über eine inotrope Potenz.

Die Erhaltung des mindestens erforderlichen mittleren arteriellen Perfusionsdrucks ist daher bei Versagen der Volumentherapie die wesentliche Indikation für Katecholamine. Eigene Ergebnisse zeigen aber, daß der massive Einsatz von Katecholaminen eine schlechte Prognose für den Patienten bedeutet. Nur ein kleiner Prozentsatz der Patienten mit mehr als einem Katecholamin in höherer Dosierung überlebt eine Sepsis/septischen Schock. Dies liegt nicht zuletzt daran, daß die peripheren Rezeptoren in einer azidotischen Stoffwechsellage vermindert auf Katecholamine ansprechen. Zudem sind die α_1 Rezeptoren in der Sepsis vermindert [45]. Es kommt dann nach einer Phase der energetisch ungünstigen Konstriktion zu einer Phase des zunehmenden Widerstandsverlustes mit Shunteröffnung bei steigenden Dosen an Katecholaminen. Der Verlust des peripheren Widerstandes muß ebenfalls als sehr ungünstiges prognostisches Kriterium angesehen werden.

Handelt es sich um einen therapierefraktären Widerstandsverlust, so ist auch der Einsatz von Angiotensin möglich, das auch bei verminderter Ansprechbarkeit auf Katecholamine noch eine Hebung des Blutdrucks bewirken kann. Inwieweit es sich hier um reine Blutdruckkosmetik handelt, ist noch nicht endgültig geklärt, aber die Zahl der Patienten, die eine Situation zur Indikation von Angiotensin überlebt haben, ist ebenfalls klein.

Eine neue therapeutische Alternative zur Stärkung der Inotropie hat sich mit den Phosphodiesterasehemmern eröffnet. Hier kommt es zu einer deutlichen Steigerung der Kontraktilität ohne die bei Katecholaminen üblichen Nebenwirkungen. Das therapeutische Prinzip stammt aus der Kardiologie und hat sich noch nicht auf allen Intensivstationen durchgesetzt. Erste eigene Erfahrungen sind aber durchaus positiv. Allerdings kann es in therapeutischer Dosierung auch zu einer hämodynamisch wirksamen Erweiterung der Peripherie kommen, die gerade in der hyperdynamen Phase nicht erwünscht ist und ein Absetzen des Medikamentes erfordert. Ebenfalls noch wenige breite Erfahrungen liegen mit dem Dopexamin vor, welches bei geringeren Nebenwirkungen die Vorteile von Dobutamin und Dopamin kombinieren soll.

Die Wahl der Flüssigkeit ist weiter umstritten. Wie bei der Initialbehandlung der Verbrennungen gibt es auch in dieser Phase „Kristallophile und Kolloidophile" [83]. Vor allem Shoemaker und Demling propagieren die Substitution mit kolloidalen Lösungen, am besten Eiweiß-Präparationen (z. B. Fresh Frozen Plasma = FFP), da hiermit die beste und physiologischste Plasmavolumenexpansion erzielt werden könne. Gleichzeitig komme es zu einer Substitution von Gerinnungsfaktoren und Albuminen. Aber auch andere kolloidale Lösungen werden wegen des kleinen, zu verabreichenden, Gesamtvolumens den kristalloiden Lösungen vorgezogen. Deren Protagonisten führen die freie Austauschbarkeit der Moleküle als Argumente ins Feld und meinen, daß das „protein rich edema" der Ausbildung eines ARDS Vorschub leistet. Hier ist die endgültige Klärung wohl noch lange nicht abgeschlossen.

Blut stellt das ideale Volumensubstitutionsmittel in der Sepsis dar. Dies wird allerdings durch die doch beträchtliche Gefahr einer Infektionsübertragung relativiert, so daß die Indikation zur Bluttransfusion streng gestellt und auf den Routineeinsatz verzichtet werden muß. Eindeutig ist die Normalisierung der Zirkulation der Schlüssel zum Therapieerfolg bei der Sepsis. Neben der hämodynamischen Stabilisierung gibt es ein ganzes Bündel flankierender Maßnahmen. Das Spektrum reicht von der als unverzichtbar geltenden Antibiotikatherapie bis zum klinisch experimentellen Einsatz neuer monoklonaler Antikörper. Einige, früher oft eingesetzte, Substanzen von fragwürdigem therapeutischem Wert wie Kortikosteroide sind dagegen heute weitgehend verlassen.

Antibiotika

Für unverzichtbar wird heute noch die Antibiotikatherapie gehalten. Unter der Vorstellung, daß nur Bakterien eine Sepsis auslösen können, war sie lange Dreh- und Angelpunkt der Sepsistherapie. Mittlerweile hat sich der Stellenwert verschoben. Natürlich ist bei einer bakteriellen Sepsis eine effiziente Antibiotikatherapie wichtig, aber es gibt Situationen in denen sie zu spät, überflüssig oder sogar schädlich sein kann [12].

Kommt die Antibiotikatherapie zu spät, so bedeutet dies, daß die „septic response" in vollem Gange ist und durch Zerstörung der Keime nicht mehr beeinflußt werden kann. Darüber hinaus kann ein bakterizider Stoß eines Antibiotikums große Mengen an Endo- und Exotoxinen freisetzen, die wiederum die „septic response" noch verstärken oder erneut ankurbeln. Border konnte zeigen, daß bei Einsatz auch multipler Antibiotika-Kombinationen zwar bestimmte Keime aus den Blutkulturen eliminiert werden, aber durch andere resistente Erreger ersetzt werden. Eine falsche Antibiotikatherapie kann zusätzlich die Resistenzentwicklung fördern, die Darmflora weiter schädigen und somit der Translokation von Enterobakterien Vorschub leisten.

Dies soll nicht bedeuten, daß auf Antibiotika verzichtet werden soll, aber es soll aufmerksam machen, Antibiotika nicht unkritisch zu geben. Vor allem muß gewarnt werden anzunehmen, daß mit einer maximalen Antibiotikatherapie unbedingt eine Wende zum Besseren eintreten muß. Dies trifft besonders auf Fälle mit systemischer Pilzinfektion zu. Setzt in solchen Situationen die Therapie zu spät ein, so muß auch bei potenten Antimykotika mit einem Therapieversagen gerechnet werden. Die Letalität generalisierter Candida Infektionen liegt in einigen Kollektiven bei fast 100 % [56], im eigenen Krankengut lag die Mortalität bei ca. 55 % [34].

Beatmung

Die Beatmung kann sehr schnell wichtiger Teil der Sepsistherapie werden, nämlich dann wenn der Patient über das Stadium der Tachypnoe ateminsuffizient wird. Eine „geplante" kontrollierte Beatmung reduziert den Energiebedarf des Patienten, vermindert die Atemarbeit und sorgt für die dringend benötigte Erhöhung der O_2-Angebots bei gleichzeitiger Vermeidung einer Hyperkapnie. Die Infusionstherapie kann kalkuliert werden, ohne daß man eine interstitielles Lungenödem fürchten muß, die Peep Beatmung ist möglicherweise sogar prophylaktisch gegen die Entwicklung eines ARDS wirksam. Der von Chirurgen oft unkritisch gefürchtete Tubus kann bei einem Sepsispatienten eine lebensrettende Maßnahme sein [91, 97].

Gerinnungssystem

Heparin ist wichtiger Bestandteil des Therapiekonzepts. Beim schweren septischen Bild kommt es häufig zu einer disseminierten intravasalen Gerinnung mit Verbrauchskoagulopathie. Ein engmaschiges Therapiemonitoring sollte hier angestrebt werden. Heparin unterbricht zwar die kausale Kette der Hyperkoagulabilität, andererseits kann es unter Therapie zu schwer kontrollierbaren Blutungen kommen.

Daher gewinnt die Substitution von Gerinnungsfaktoren immer mehr an klinischer Bedeutung. Gründe dafür sind die zunehmenden Erkenntnisse über Mitbeteiligung des Gerinnungssystems in der Sepsis und die wesentlich für die Gewebsazidose verantwortlichen Mikrozirkulationsstörungen u.a. auch durch disseminierte Mikrothrombosierung. Eine Schlüsselrolle spielt hier das AT III (Heparin Kofaktor). Es unterbricht sowohl die Bildung von Fibrin über die aktivierten Faktoren XIIa-X auf jeder Stufe als auch die Kallikreinaktivierung über die der Komplementfaktor C1 aktiviert werden kann [78]. Die Wirkung des Heparin ohne ausreichenden Spiegel an ATIII ist erheblich eingeschränkt. Neben der Zuführung als Einzelkomponente hat sich die Applikation von FFP in der Klinik bewährt. Neben dem volumenexpandierenden Effekt des FFP werden auch plasmatische Gerinnungsfaktoren, Proteinaseinhibitoren und AT III substituiert. Die untere Interventionsgrenze für AT III ist noch nicht exakt definiert, liegt aber in den meisten Abteilungen zwischen 75% – 50% der Normaktivität [95].

Kortikosteroide

Der Einsatz von Kortikosteroiden bildet periodisch ein Diskussionsthema. Bis vor kurzem gab es erstaunlicherweise kaum Studien über die Wirksamkeit des Kortisons bei der Sepsis. Die Ergebnisse der Veterans Administration Sepsis Study (VA) und anderer Studien zeigen eindeutig, daß Kortison in der Sepsis trotz einer oft beboachteten temporären klinischen Besserung keine Verbesserung der Überlebensrate bringt [92]. Die Rate an Sekundärinfektionen war im Vergleich zur Kontrollgruppe sogar höher [86]. Dies steht im Widerspruch zu vielen tierexperimentellen Ergebnissen, aber hier wurde meist ein „pretreatment" durchgeführt oder das Kortison so früh appliziert, wie dies in der klinischen Situation kaum möglich ist. Die Wirkung scheint prinzipiell vorhanden, offenbar aber sehr vom Zeitpunkt der Applikation abhängig zu sein. Nach den heute gewonnenen klinischen Daten ist einer Anwendung von Kortison im septischen Schock eher skeptisch gegenüberzustehen [16, 52, 101].

Opiatantagonisten

Ein weitere fragwürdige Medikamentengruppe sind die Opiatantagonisten (z. B. Naloxon). Es ist aus experimentellen und klinischen Untersuchungen bekannt, daß Opiatantagonisten die Wirkungen körpereigener Enkephaline und Endorphine aufheben und damit z B. vorübergehend einen peripheren Widerstandsverlust auffangen können. Aber ähnlich wie bei Kortikosteroiden hat sich in der Klinik keine signifikante Verbesserung der Überlebensrate feststellen lassen. Dies ist möglicherweise aber auch in den bisher verwandten niedrigen Dosierungen begründet, so daß hier zukünftig noch mit neuen Entwicklungen zu rechnen ist [46].

Immunglobuline – Monoklonale Antikörper

Ein ewig aktuelles Diskussionsthema ist die Anwendung von Immunglobulinen. Frühere klinische Versuche ergaben keinen lebensrettenden Effekt der Immunglobuline, was auch an der Zusammensetzung der Präparate gelegen haben mag. Im eigenen Kollektiv war die prophylaktische Applikation eines Pseudomonasspezifischen Immunglobulins nicht in der Lage die infektiösen Komplikationen signifikant zu senken. Die Ergebnisse einer therapeutischen kontrollierten, randomisierten Doppelblindstudie stehen noch aus [89, 90]. Neuere Untersuchungen haben jedoch zeigen können, daß eine frühe Administration von Ig Präparationen mit hohem IgM Anteil einen Effekt auf die Mortalitätsrate haben [71]. Den IgM Fraktionen wird ein ähnlicher Toxin-eliminierender Effekt zugeschrieben wie den monoklonalen Antikörpern. Entscheidend ist offensichtlich auch hier der Zeitpunkt der Applikation, der vor einer irreversiblen Perpetuierung der pathophysiologischen Reaktionskette liegen muß. Eine mögliche therapeutische Alternative besteht in der Immunisierung mit sog. „rauhen Mutanten", die eine Abmilderung der toxischen Wirkungen verwandter Stämme bewirken [6].

Viele Hoffnungen konzentrieren sich derzeit auf den klinischen Einsatz monoklonaler Antikörper gegen Endotoxin und TNF α, die sich im Experiment bereits bewährt haben [35, 100]. Aus dem klinischen Bereich liegen erste Ergebnisse einer multizentrischen Studie über den Einsatz eines humanen Endotoxin Antikörpers (HA-1A) bei gram-negativer Sepsis vor. Bei Patienten mit Bakteriämie zeigte der MAK eine signifikante Reduktion der sepsisbedingten Mortalität, während bei septischen Patienten ohne Bakteriämie kein signifikanter Effekt auszumachen war [105]. Erste eigene Erfahrungen mit dem Einsatz des mittlerweile kommerziell erhältlichen Antikörpers waren durchaus positiv. Für den MAK gilt ähnliches wie für Antibiotika oder Ig bezüglich des Zeitpunkts der Applikation. Hemmschwelle ist in diesem Fall sicher der hohe Preis der Therapie (ca DM 6000.-). Allerdings werden bei erfolgreichem Einsatz die Therapiefolgekosten deutlich reduziert und möglicherweise durch erhebliche Einsparungen im Bereich Plasmaersatzmittel, Katecholamine und Antibiotika ausgeglichen.

Das Prinzip des Anti-TNF beruht auf der Blockade eines finalen Mediators, der viele der Endotoxineffekte letztlich moduliert. Der klinische Effekt könnte dem

HA-1A MAK ähneln, würde natürlich aber viele physiologische Reaktionen ebenfalls blockieren. Geht man davon aus, daß das körpereigene Immunsystem in dieser Situation überstimuliert ist, so werden möglicherweise nur die autoaggressiv wirkenden Spitzen abgebrochen. Hier liegen zum jetzigen Zeitpunkt noch wenige allgemein gültige Empfehlungen vor, erste Berichte sind aber ermutigend.

Sonstige Substanzen

Im experimentellen Stadium bzw. in der Phase des klinischen Versuchs befinden sich derzeit eine Reihe von Substanzen mit sehr unterschiedlichen Angriffspunkten. Dazu gehören Zyklo- und Lipooxygenaseblocker, O_2-Radikalenfänger und Hypoxanthinantagonisten, IL 2 Rezeptorantagonisten und monoklonale Antikörper gegen Endotoxin (LPA) und TNF bzw. Pseudomonaden. Ibuprofen hat sich im Experiment als potenter Zyklooxygenasehemmer erwiesen, ebenso Indomethacin. Sowohl hämodynamische Parameter als auch die Ausbildung eines extravasalen Ödems waren deutlich besser als in der Kontrollgruppe. Ibuprofen führt außerdem im Gegensatz zu Indomethacin nicht zu einer gleichzeitigen Stimulierung der Lipooxygenase [13]. In einer ersten klinischen Studie konnten diese Ergebnisse allerdings nicht in dieser Deutlichkeit nachvollzogen werden [42].

Zyklooxygenase und Lipooxygenasehemmer haben sich in vielen Experimenten als wirksam erwiesen, die Effekte der traumatisch stimulierten Produktion von Eicosanoiden wie Thromboxan (TX), PG E2 und Leukotrienen (LT B4, LT C4) zu mildern. Keine Schockform setzt so viel Eicosanoide frei wie die Sepsis [65]. Viele experimentelle Untersuchungen lassen aber durch prätraumatische Medikamentenapplikation keine klinischen Analogieschlüsse zu. Die Gabe von O_2 Scavengern wie SOD oder Katalase hat sich ebenfalls im Experiment, aber auch in einigen klinischen Situationen bewährt, ebenso Allupurinol als Blocker der Xanthinoxydase. Aus der Analyse der publizierten Arbeiten ergibt sich auch hier als limitierender Faktor für den Effekt der Zeitpunkt der Applikation. Ein günstiger Effekt ist nahezu immer bei früher Gabe der Substanzen zu beobachten, bei in Gang gekommener Reaktionskette ist das Geschehen kaum noch aufzuhalten.

Die Zukunft der Sepsistherapie liegt sicher in der Unterstützung bzw. Beeinflussung des Immunsystems. Dazu gehören sowohl die Stimulation abwehrstärkender Mechanismen als auch die Blockade schädigender Effekte. Zu diesen neuen Therapieformen, die sich alle noch im Stadium des klinischen Experiments befinden, gehört der Einsatz von rekombinantem IL 2. Im Tierexperiment senkte die Kombination mit Indomethacin die Letalität des septischen Schocks von 66 auf 38 % [47]. Auch die Behandlung mit GCSF (granulocyte colony stimulating factor) zur Produktions- und Differenzierungssteigerung neutrophiler Granulozyten oder die Applikation von y-IFN zur Verbesserung der Makrophagenfunktion, Antigenpräsentation und Steigerung der IL 1 Synthese steht derzeit in der klinischen Prüfungsphase bei Schwerverbrannten [30].

Organversagen

Trotz des Einsatzes aller intensivmedizinischen Mittel gelingt es oft nicht die Ausbildung eines Organversagen zu verhindern. Die klinischen Anzeichen sind Funktionseinschränkungen als Folge der Hypoperfusion. Laborchemisch zeigen alle Organe spezifische Veränderungen. Außer der pharmakologischen Unterstützung und in einigen Zentren auch mechanischer Pumpunterstützung des Herzens und der Möglichkeit der Dialyse in allen Formen, gibt es leider kaum Möglichkeiten die Funktionen der betroffenen Organsysteme außer durch Verbesserung der energetischen Situation gezielt zu verbessern.

Das akute Nierenversagen (ANV) gehörte noch vor 20 Jahren zu den unbedingt letalen Komplikationen. Durch die Möglichkeiten der Dialyse gelingt es heute vielfach Phasen der Niereninsuffizienz zu überbrücken. Dennoch haben septische Krankheitsbilder mit OV bei Mitbeteiligung der Niere auch heute noch die schlechteste Prognose aller MOV Kombinationen. Dies liegt möglicherweise weniger an der ersetzten exkretorischen Funktion, als an der nicht kompensierten sekretorischen Funktion der Niere. Welches Verfahren zur Dialyse gewählt wird, hängt nur von den lokalen Gegebenheiten ab. In jedem Fall ist aber die Kinetik der verabreichten Antibiotika und anderer Medikamente zu beachten, die bei unterschiedlichen Verfahren verschieden beeinflußt werden. In erfahrenen Händen erzielen alle gebräuchlichen Verfahren gute klinische Resultate.

Alle anderen Organsysteme sind derzeit nur indirekt beeinflußbar. Wichtigstes Prinzip ist die eingangs erwähnte Besserung der Perfusion und damit der Oxygenierung. Spezielle auf Organschäden abgestimmte Infusionskonzepte halten einer kritischen Betrachtung für den Intensivpatienten nicht stand. Dennoch sollte z. B. bei beginnendem oder manifestem Leberversagen auf die Applikation hepato-toxischer Substanzen verzichtet werden. Ähnliches gilt bei der Niere z. B. für nephro-toxische Antibiotika und Antimykotika.

Ernährung

Ein wichtiger Faktor, nicht nur in der Prävention sondern auch bei manifester Sepsis ist die Ernährung des Patienten. Der Immunstatus des Patienten ist eng mit seinem Ernährungsstatus verknüpft. Dabei ist besonders in der Sepsis auf die Zusammensetzung der Energieträger zu achten. Eine ausreichende enterale Ernährung sichert z. B. nicht nur die Energiezufuhr sondern auch die Integrität der Darmmukosa und verhindert möglicherweise die die Sepsis unterhaltende Translokation [25, 31]. Dies kann durch parenterale Substitution in dieser Form nicht erreicht werden. Wichtig ist auch die zusätzliche Substitution von Vitaminen und Mineralien, deren Umsatz in der Sepsis gesteigert ist [19, 61].

Monitoring

Wichtig für den Erfolg beim Einsatz aller beschriebenen Therapieformen ist eine suffiziente Steuerung der Therapie. Die polypragmatische Anwendung aller „guten" Substanzen und Maßnahmen verlangt eine engmaschige Kontrolle der physiologischen und laborchemischen Parameter. Dies kann durchaus in Stufen erfolgen, da ein Patient, der z.B. die Kriterien der Sepsis erfüllt, noch nicht in jedem Fall ein maximales Monitoring benötigt. So werden in der ersten Stufe ein zentraler Venenkatheter, Urinkatheter und im Fall der Beatmung ein arterieller Zugang sicher ausreichen. Bei kritischer, vital bedrohlicher, Situation ist dagegen die Plazierung eines Pulmonaliskatheters und als zentralen Zugang die Insertion eines Bi-Lumenkatheters zu empfehlen. Ergebnisse von Waxmann zeigen, daß die klinischen Vitalparameter nur in der Hälfte aller Fälle die tatsächliche physiologische Situation exakt wiedergeben. So wird z. B. bei steigendem Venendruck eher Volumen eingespart, der Patient kann aber in der gleichen Situation diese hohe Vorlast brauchen. Aus dieser Situation läßt sich auch nicht ablesen, ob wirklich eine hohe Rechtsbelastung bzw. Rechtsinsuffizienz oder ein hoher pulmonaler Widerstand vorliegt. Zur Steuerung der Volumentherapie und Titrierung z. B. der Katecholamintherapie erscheint in diesen Fällen die Nutzung eines Pulmonalvenenkatheters, beschränkt auf die vital bedrohliche Phase, unbedingt indiziert [99].

Drug monitoring sollte, soweit möglich, für Antibiotika betrieben werden. Gerade bei Verbrannten mit großen Körperwasserverlusten über verbrannte Oberflächen und/oder eingeschränkter Nierenfunktion sollte der Serumspiegel häufiger kontrolliert werden. Urinkatheter und Magensonde sind selbstverständlich und bedürfen keiner weiteren Erläuterung. An Laborparametern sollten die Gerinnungsparameter, Laktat als Stoffwechseläquivalent und die Nieren- und Leberfunktionswerte engmaschig bestimmt werden. Ein interessantes Konzept ist die Überwachung der intestinalen Stoffwechselsituation durch die intraluminale Tonometrie, die durch Erfassung der H_2 Konzentration einen Überblick über eine Gewebsazidose und damit eine Minderperfusion erlaubt [32].

Prävention

Prävention ist sicher die beste Therapie der Sepsis. Dieser in sich widersprüchliche Satz sollte dennoch als Leitmotiv über der Behandlung des septischen Patienten stehen. Die noch immer hohe Letalität dieser Patienten, selbst unter Einsatz modernster Therapiekonzepte, macht deutlich, daß Prävention durch Exzision verbrannter Areale und schnelle Deckung durch autologe Haut, Infektverhütung durch Unterbrechung der Kontaminationskette, strikte Hygiene am Patienten [22, 102] und restriktive Antibiotikapolitik die wichtigsten Pfeiler der Therapie sind [22, 23, 53]. Schlüssel und wichtigster Punkt ist sicher die schnelle, möglichst unblutige Operation, mit der Beseitigung avitaler Gewebe, die ja auch ohne bakterielle Besiedlung ein septisches Geschehen auslösen können.

Die klinische Bewährungsprobe bestanden hat die enterale und topische Pilzprophylaxe. Im eigenen Kollektiv konnten die Rate systemischer Candida Infektionen durch konsequente Prophylaxe signifikant gesenkt werden [34]. Andere Gruppen berichten über eine deutliche Senkung der Infektionsmorbidität nach Polytrauma oder Herzoperationen durch die selektive Darm Dekontamination (SDD). Inwieweit diese Ergebnisse auf Verbrennungseinheiten übertragen werden können, bleibt laufenden klinischen Studien vorbehalten [41, 88].

Von entscheidender Bedeutung ist die personelle und apparative Kapazität der Verbrennungszentren. Geringe personelle Ausstattung, sowohl im chirurgischen wie im anästhesiologischen Bereich, bei oberflächlicher Betrachtung ein Kostenspareffekt, bedeutet eine kleinere Zahl betreuender und damit Patienten operierender Ärzte. Dies führt zwangsläufig zu einer Verlängerung der OP-Zeiten, Verschieben von Operationen und höherer Sepsisinzidenz mit Verlängerung des stationären Aufenthaltes. Die dadurch entstehenden Kosten können sich bei einem Patienten schnell zu der Größenordnung eines Jahresgehaltes eines Assistenzarztes aufsummieren.

Betrachtet man die Tagessätze in Verbrennungszentren, so liegen diese zwischen 2300–5600.- DM. Eine komplikationsbedingte Therapieverlängerung um 30 Tage bedeutet z. B. maximale Mehrkosten von DM 150.000.-! Gerade die Kosten-Nutzen-Analyse wird in der Zukunft bei Therapiekonzepten häufiger gefragt sein, d. h. die eingesetzten Mittel werden auf ihre Effizienz geprüft. Bei den enormen Kosten in der Intensivtherapie werden unsere Maßnahmen am ultimativen Erfolg, dem Überleben des Patienten gemessen. Ein rationeller, und vor allem zeitgerechter Einsatz unserer therapeutischen Möglichkeiten ist daher auch im Sinne des wachsenden Kostendruckkes wichtig und unabdingbar.

Hierzu gehört aber auch neben der ärztlichen Ausstattung die Besetzung des gesamten Verbrennungs-Teams. Der Einsatz von Physio- und Ergotherapie kann nirgends so intensiv ausgeübt werden wie in der Verbrennungseinheit selbst. Strebt man eine frühe Rehabilitation und Reintegration des Verbrannten an, so muß diese Therapie eher intensiviert als abgebaut werden. Die zunächst höheren Personalkosten werden durch eine Verkürzung der Rehabilitations- und Krankenhausphase mehrfach kompensiert.

Literatur

1. Abraham E (1991) Physiologic stress and cellular ischemia: relationship to immunosuppression and susceptibility to sepsis. Crit Care Med 19(5):613–622
2. Ayres SM (1986) Sepsis and septic shock – A synthesis of ideas and proposals for the direction of future research. In: Sibbald WJ, Sprung CL (eds) New Horizons: Perspectives on Sepsis and septic shock. Fullerton, Society of Critical Care Medicine, pp 375–392
3. Basadre JO, Traber DL, Traber LD, Herndon DN (1990) Systemic mediators of endotoxemia in a neutropenic animal model. Crit Care Med 18(4):282
4. Baue AE (1975) Multiple, progressive, or sequential systems failure. Arch Surg 110:779–781
5. Baue AE (1989) Zelluläre und subzelluläre Funktionen der vitalen Organe bei Sepsis und Multiorganversagen. In: Reinhart K, Eyrich K (Hrsg) Sepsis. Springer, Berlin, pp 176–197
6. Baumgartner JD, Glauser MP (1989) Immuntherapie und Immunprophylaxe bei Sepsis. In: Reinhart K, Eyrich K (Hrsg.) Sepsis. Springer, Berlin, pp 350–361
7. Berg S, Jannsoon I, Lauzent TC, Walther S, Hesselvik JF (1990) High serum hyaluronan in porcine sepsis – Relation to hypotension. Crit Care Med 18(4):263 (Abstract)
8. Bergmann U, König W, Gross-Weege W, Schlüter B, Köller M, Erbs G, Müller FE (1990) Basophil releasability in severely burned patients. J Trauma 30(11):1372–1379
9. Bernstein A, Fox G, Neal A, Rutledge F, Sibbald W (1990) The effect of exogenous symphatimimetics on coronary vasodilatory reserve and 02 metabolism in hyperdynamic sepsis. Crit Care Med 18(4):181 (Abstract)
10. Bone RC (1991) Let's agree on terminology: Definition of Sepsis. Crit Care Med 19(7):973–976
11. Bone RC, Fisher CJ, Clemmer TP, Slotman GJ, Metz CA, Balk RA, Methylprednisolon Sever Sepsis Study Group (1989) Sepsis syndrome: A valid clinical entity. Crit Care Med 17(5):389–393
12. Border JR, Hassett J, Laduca J, Seibel R, Steinberg S, Mills B, Losi P, Border D (1987) The gut origin septic states in blunt multiple trauma (ISS=40) in the ICU. Ann Surg 206(4):427–448
13. Byrne K, Careay PD, Sielaff TD, Jenkins JK, Blocher CR, Cooper KR, Fowler AA, Sugerman HJ (1991) Ibuprofen prevents deterioration in static transpulmonary compliance and transalveolar protein flux in septic porcine acute lung injury. J Trauma 31(2):155–166
14. Cain MS, Curtis CE (1991) Experimental models of pathologic oxygen supply dependency. Crit Care Med 19(5):603–612

15. Cain SM (1989) Mechanismen des eingeschränkten Sauerstoffangebots bei Sepsis und ARDS. In: Reinhart K, Eyrich K Sepsis. Springer, Berlin, pp 153–161
16. Carrico CJ, Meakins JL, Marshall JC (1986) Multiple organ failure syndrome. Arch Surg 121:196–208
17. Carvajal HF, Feinstein R, Traber DL, Parks DH, Kiker R, Larson DL, Whorton EB (1981) An objective method for early diagnosis of gram-negative septicemia in burned children. J Trauma 21(4):221–227
18. Cerami A, Beutler B (1988) The role of cachectin/TNF in endotoxic shock and cachexia. Immunol Tod 9(1):28–31
19. Cerra FB (1989) Ernährungstherapie bei Sepsis: Gesichertes und Perspektiven. In: Reinhart K, Eyrich K Sepsis. Springer, Berlin, pp 261–268
20. Clowes GHA (1974) Pulmonary abnormalities in sepsis. Surg Clin North Amer 54(5):993–1013
21. Danner RL, Suffredini AF, Van Dervort AL, Ceska M, Stuetz PL, Zablotny JA (1990) Neutrophil activating peptide-1/Interleukin 8 concentrations in human septic shock. Crit Care Med 18(4):281 (Abstract)
22. Daschner FD (1985) Nosocomial infections in intensive care units. Intensive Care Med 11:284–291
23. Daschner FD, Kappstein I (1989) Nützliche und nutzlose Maßnahmen zur Verhinderung von Infektionen und Sepsis bei Intensivpatienten. In: Reinhart K, Eyrich K Sepsis. Springer, Berlin, pp 66–81
24. DeCamp MM, Demling RH (1988) Posttraumatic multisystem organ failure. Jama 260(4):530–534
25. Deitch EA, Specian RD, Berg RD (1991) Endotoxin induced bacterial translocation and mucosal permeability: Role of xanthin oxyclase, complement activation, and macrophage products. Crit Care Med 19(6):185–191
26. Demling RH, LaLonde C (1989) Burn Trauma. Thieme, New York
27. Eickacker PQ, Hoffman WD, Kuo G, Richmond S, Banks SM, MacVittie T, Natanson C (1990) Tumor necrosis factor but not Interleukin-1 induces sustained but reversible Hypoxemia, Alveolar protein and neutrophil accumulation, and hemodynamic depression in dogs. Crit Care Med 18(4):280 (Abstract)
28. Eiseman B, Beart R, Norton L (1977) Multiple organ failure. Surg Gyn Obst 144(3):323–326
29. Erdmann E, Reuschel-Janetschek E (1989) Hämodynamik in der Sepsis und im septischen Schock. Intensivmed 26(1):16–21
30. Faist E, Storck M, Ertel W, Mewes A, v. Donnersmarck H (1989) Suppression der zellvermittelten Immunität nach schweren Brand- und Mehrfachverletzungen. Intensivmed 26(1):102–110
31. Fiddian-Green RG, Baker S (1991) Nosocomial pneumonia in the critically ill: Product of aspiration or translocation. Crit Care Med 19(6):763–769
32. Fink MP (1991) Gastrointestinal mucosal injury in experimental models of shock, trauma, and sepsis. Crit Care Med 19(5):627–641
33. Fry DE, Pearlstein L, Fulton RL, Polk HC (1980) Multiple system organ failure. Arch Surg 115:136–140
34. Germann G, Janshof G, Steinau HU (1992) Incidence and Sequence of Sepsis and Multiple Organ Failure (MOF) in Severely Burned Patients. ABA 24th:Annual Meeting-1.-4.4.92
35. Gorelick KJ, Wedel NI, Kunz AY, Wilson KM, Greenberg RN (1990) E5 antiendotoxin antibody in gramnegative sepsis: report of phase II study. Crit Care Med 18(4):260 (Abstract)
36. Goris JA (1987) Pathophysiology of multiple organ failure with „sepsis". Med Klin 82:546–547
37. Goris RJA, Boekholtz WKF, van Bebber IPT, Nuytinck JKS, Schillings PHM (1986) Multiple-Organ failure and sepsis without bacteria. Arch Surg 121(8):897–901
38. Goris RJA, Nuytinck HKS, Redl H (1987) Scoring systems and predictors of ARDS and MOF. In: Schlag G, Redl H Progress in clinical and biological research – Monitoring and treatment of shock – First Vienna shock forum. Alan R. Liss, New York, pp 3–15
39. Gramm HJ, Reinhart K, Goecke J, v. Bülow J (1989) Symptome und Befunde zur Frühdiagnose des Sepsissyndrom. In: Reinhart K, Eyrich K Sepsis. Springer, Berlin, pp 53–65
40. Gutierrez G (1991) Cellular energy metabolism during hypoxia. Crit Care Med 19(5):619–626

41. Hartenauer U, Thülig B, Lawin P, Fegeler W (1990) Selective Decontamination of the digestive tract (SDD) in cardio-thoracic surgery patients. Crit Care Med 18(4):206 (Abstract)
42. Haupt MT, Jastremski MS, Clemmer TP, Metz CA, Goris GB (1991) Effect of ibuprofen in patients with severe sepsis: A randomized, double-blind, multicenter study. Crit Care Med 19(11):1339–1347
43. Hersh M, Groom A, Sibbald W (1990) Morphometrical quantitated capillary dilation fails to prevent myocardial cellular necrosis in a normotensive hyperdynamic septic model. Crit Care Med 18(4):181 (Abstract)
44. Hesselvik JF, Blomback M, Brodin B, Maller R (1989) Coagulation, fibrinolysis, and kallikrein systems in sepsis: relation to outcome. Crit Care Med 17(8):724–733
45. Higgins TL, Chernow B (1989) Neue Konzepte bei der pharmakologischen Behandlung des Herz-Kreislauf-Versagens im septischen Schock. In: Reinhart K, Eyrich K (Hrsg.) Sepsis. Springer, Berlin, pp 414–423
46. Holaday JW (1989) Die Bedeutung der Opiatantagonisten bei der Behandlung des septischen Schocks. In: Reinhart K, Eyrich K (Hrsg.) Sepsis. Springer, Berlin, pp 401–413
47. Horgan PG; Mannick JA, Dubravec DB, Rodrick ML (1990) Effect of low dose recombinant interleukin 2 plus indomethacin on mortality after sepsis in a murine burn model. Br J Surg 77:401–404
48. Jochum M, Fritz H, Nast-Kolb D, Inthorn D (1990) Granulozyten-Elastase als prognostischer Parameter. Deutsches Ärzteblatt 87(19):1526–1533
49. Jordan DA, Miller CF, Kubos KL, Rogers MC (1987) Evaluation of sepsis in a critically ill surgical population. Crit Care Med 15(10):897–904
50. Knaus WA, Draper EA, Wagner DP, Zimmermann JE (1985) APACHE II:A severity of disease classification system. Crit Care Med 13(10):818–829
51. Köller M, König W (1991) Immunopathophysiologie des Verbrennungstraumas. DMW 116:67–73
52. Kreger BE, Craven DE, Carling PC, McCabe WR (1980) Gram-negative bacteremia. Amer J Med 68:332–343
53. MacMillan BG (1981) The control of burn wound sepsis. Intensive Care Med 7:63–69
54. Marshall JC, Christou NV, Horn R, Meakins JL (1988) The microbiology of multiple organ failure. Arch Surg 123:309–315
55. Marshall WG, Dimick AR (1983) The natural history of major burns with multiple subsystem failure. J Trauma 23(2):102–105
56. Martich GD, Cunnion RE, Ognibene FP, Suffredini AF, Parker MM (1990) Candidemic septic shock in comparison to bacteremic shock: Serial hemodynamics and outcome. Crit Care Med 18(4):263 (Abstract)
57. Mason AD, McManus AT, Pruitt BA (1986) Association of burn mortality and Bacteremia – A 25 year review. Arch Surg 121:1027–1031
58. Merrell SW, Saffle JR, Larson CM, Sullivan JJ (1989) The declining incidence of fatal sepsis following thermal injury. J Trauma 29(10):1362–1365
59. Meßmer K, Kreimeier U, Hammersen F (1989) Sepsis, In: Reinhart K, Eyrich K Veränderungen im Bereich der Mikrozirkulation bei Sepsis und septischem Schock. Springer, Berlin, pp 163–175
60. Mitsuo T, Tnaka H, Ikegami K, Watanabe K, Yukioka T, Shimazaki S, Matsuda H (1990) Right ventricular dysfunction in septic patients. Crit Care Med 18(4):181–192 (Abstract)
61. Moyer E, Cerra F, Chenier R, Peters D, Oswald G, Watson F, Yu L, Mcmenamy RH, Border JR (1981) Multiple systems organ failure: VI. Death predictors in the trauma-septic-state - The most critical determinants. J Trauma 21(10):862–869
62. Müller U, Hallström S, Koidl B, Schlage G, Werdan K (1989) Wirkung einer kardiodepressiven Fraktion (CDF) aus dem Plasma von Hunden im Shock in Herzmuskelzellkulturen. Intensivmed 26(1):45–49
63. Neuhof H (1989) Zur Rolle der Mediatoren bei der Sepsis. Intensivmed 26(1):3–9
64. Nuytinck JKS, Goris JA, Redl H, Schlag G, van Munster PJJ (1986) Posttraumatic complications and inflammatory mediators. Arch Surg 121:886–890
65. Oettinger W, Berger D, Beger HG (1989) Klinische Relevanz von Endotoxin und Eicosanoiden bei schwerer Sepsis. In: Reinhart K, Eyrich K (Hrsg.) Sepsis. Springer, Berlin, pp 329–338

66. Parillo JE, Parker MM, Natanson C, Suffredini AF, Danner RL, Cunnion RE, Ognibene FP (1990) Septic shock in humans. Ann Int Med 113(3):227–242
67. Parker MM, Parillo JE (1989) Sepsis und Herzfunktion. In: Reinhart K, Eyrich K (Hrsg) Sepsis. Springer, Berlin, pp 124–136
68. Pilz G, Werdan K (1989) Score-Systeme bei Sepsis und septischem Schock: Diagnosestellung, Verlaufsbeurteilung und Therapiekontrolle. Intensivmed 26(1):65–71
69. Redl H, Sclag G, Goris JA, Pacher R (1989) Scoresysteme in der Intensivmedizin. Intensivmed 26(1):60–64
70. Reinhart K (1989) Sauerstofftransport und Gewebeoxygenierung bei Sepsis und septischem Schock. In: Reinhart K, Eyrich K (Hrsg.) Sepsis. Springer, Berlin, pp 137–152
71. Schedel I, Dreikhausen U, Nentwig B, Höckenschnieder M, Rauthmann D, Balikcioglu S, Coldewy R, Deicher H (1991) Treatment of Gram-negativ septic shock with an immunoglobulin preparation: A prospective, randomized clinical trial. Crit Care Med 19(9):1104–1113
72. Schlüter B, König W (1990) Microbial pathogenicity and host defense mechanisms – crucial parameters of posttraumatic infections. Thorac Cardiovasc Surgeon 38:339–347
73. Schlüter B, König W, Köller M, Erbs G, Müller FE (1990) Studies on B-lymphozyte dysfunctions in severely burned patients. J Trauma 30(119):1380–1389
74. Schottmüller H (1914) Wesen und Behandlung der Sepsis. Verh Dtsch Ges Inn Med 31:257–276
75. Schultze-Osthoff K, Fiers W (1991) Die Rolle des Tumor-Nekrose-Faktors im septischen Schock. Gelbe Hefte XXXI:61–67
76. Schuster HP (1989) Sepsis – Klinische Definition und Inzidenz. In: Reinhart K, Eyrich K (Hrsg.) Sepsis. Springer, Berlin, pp 1–7
77. Schuster HP (1989) Sepsis als Ursache des Multiorganversagens Definition, Pathophysiologie und diagnostische Parameter. Anaesth Intensivther Notfallmed 24:206–211
78. Seitz R, Wolf M, Egbring R, Havemann K (1989) The disturbance of hemostasis in septic shock: role of neutrophil elastase and thrombin, effects of antithrombin III and plasma substitution. Eur J Haematol 43:22–28
79. Sheagren JN (1989) Pathophysiologie der Sepsis und des septischen Schocks. In: Reinhart K, Eyrich K (Hrsg.) Sepsis. Springer, Berlin, pp 26–40
80. Shoemaker WC (1987) Circulatory mechanisms of shock and their mediators. Crit Care Med 15(8):787–794
81. Shoemaker WC, Appel PL, Kram HB (1988) Tissue oxygen debt as a determinant of lethal and nonlethal postoperative organ failure. Crit Care Med 16(11):1117–1120
82. Shoemaker WC, Appel PL, Kram HB (1991) Oxygen transport measurement to evaluate tissue perfusion and titrate therapy: dobutamine and dopamine effects. Crit Care Med 19(5):672–688
83. Sibbald WJ, Marshall J, Christou N, Girotti M, McCormack D, Rostein O, Martin C, Meakins J (1991) "Sepsis" – Clarity of existing terminology... or more confusion? Crit Care Med 19(8):996–998
84. Sibbald WJ, Raper RF, Bersten AD (1989) Kreislaufveränderungen beim septischen Syndrom. In: Reinhart K, Eyrich K (Hrsg.) Sepsis. Springer, Berlin, pp 108–123
85. Sprung CL (1991) Definition of Sepsis – Have we reached a consensus? Crit Care Med 19(7):849–851
86. Sprung CL, Schrein RMH, Long WM (1989) Kortikosteroide und nicht steroidale antiinflammatorische Substanzen beim Sepsissyndrom. In: Reinhart K, Eyrich K (Hrsg.) Sepsis. Springer, Berlin, pp 97–107
87. Sprung CL, Schultz DR, Marcial E, Caralis PV, Gelbard MA, Arnold PI, Long WI (1986) Complement activation in septic shock patients. Crit Care Med 14(6):525–528
88. Stouenbeek CP, van Saene HKF, Miranda DR, Zandstra DF (1984) The effect of selective decontamination of the digestive tract on colonization and infection rate in multiple trauma patients. Intensive Care Med 10:185–192
89. Stuttmann R, Hartert M, Coleman JE, Kill H, Germann G, Doehn M (1989) Prophylaxe mit einem Pseudomonas-Immunoglobulin bei Brandverletzten. Intensivmed 26(1):130–137
90. Stuttmann R, Vogt C, Hartert M, Knüttgen D, Germann G, Doehn M (1989) Supportive Therapie des septischen Schocks mit Pseudomonas-Immunglobulinen. Intensivmed 26(1):124–129

91. Suter PM (1989) Behandlungsmöglichkeiten des akuten Atemnotsyndroms (ARDS) bei Sepsis. In: Reinhart K, Eyrich K (Hrsg.) Sepsis. Springer, Berlin, pp 91–96
92. The Veterans Administration systemic sepsis cooperative study group (1987) Effect of high-dose glucocorticoid therapy on mortality in patients with clinical signs of systemic sepsis. New Engl J Med 317:659–665
93. Till GO (1991) Oxygen radical – mediated injury. 2. Int. Congress on the Immune Consequences of Trauma, Shock, and Sepsis 2 (Abstract)
94. Vespasiano MC, Zimmermann JJ, Lewandowski JR (1990) Longitudinal analysis of polymorphonuclear leukocyte superoxide anion generation in adults with septic shock. Crit Care Med 18(4):283 (Abstract)
95. Vogel GE (1986) The patient in shock – Clinical picture and pathophysiology. Endoscopy 18:1–5
96. Wagenknecht B, Hug M, Hübner G, Werdan K (1989) Myokardiale Wirkung von Mediatoren. Intensivmed 26(1):32–40
97. Wardle EN (1984) Shock lungs: The post-traumatic respiratory distress syndrome. Quart J Med 211:317–329
98. Watters JM, Wilmore DW (1989) Metabolische Veränderungen bei Sepsis und septischem Schock. In: Reinhart K, Eyrich K (Hrsg.) Sepsis. Springer, Berlin, pp 379–400
99. Waxman K, Fries DJ (1991) Adequate resuscitation of burn patients may not be measured by urine output and vital signs. Crit Care Med 19(3):327–329
100. Wedel NI, Gorelick KJ, Saria EA, Weidler DJ, Blaschke TF (1990) Pharmacokinetics and safety of antiendotoxin antibodies E5 in normal subjects. Crit Care Med 18(4):213 (Abstract)
101. Weigel JA, Norcross JF, Bormann KR, Sayder WH (1985) Early steroid therapy for respiratory failure. Arch Surg 120:536–541
102. Wenzel RP, Thompson RL, Landry SM, Russel BS, Miller PJ, Ponce de Leon S, Miller GB (1983) Hospital acquired infections in intensive care unit patients: an overview with emphasis in epidemics. Infect Control 4:371–382
103. Wilson RF (1989) Prävention und Therapie der Sepsis bei operativen Risikopatienten. In: Reinhart K, Eyrich K (Hrsg.) Sepsis. Springer, Berlin, pp 269–313
104. Yuesheng H, Ao L, Zongcheng Y (1992) A prospective clinical study on the pathogenesis of multiple organ failure in severely burned patients. Burns 18(1):30–34
105. Ziegler EJ, Fisher CH, Sprung CL et al. (1991) Treatment of Gram-negative bacteremia and septic shock with HA-1A human monoclonal antibody against endotoxin. N Engl J Med 324:429–437
106. Zimmermann JJ (1989) Sepsis and Leukozytenfunktion – Schaden und Nutzen. In: Reinhart K, Eyrich K (Hrsg.) Sepsis. Springer, Berlin, pp 198–221

Anschrift des Verfassers:
Priv. Doz. Dr. G. Germann
BG Unfallklinik Ludwigshafen
Abt. für Verbrennungen, Plastische- und Handchirurgie
Ludwig-Guttmann-Str. 13
D-67071 Ludwigshafen-Oggersheim

E. **Fritze,** Bochum (Hrsg.)
unter Mitarbeit von Burkard **May,** Bochum

Die ärztliche Begutachtung

Rechtsfragen, Funktionsprüfungen, Beurteilungen, Beispiele

1992. 4., vollständig neu bearbeitete und erweiterte Auflage.
979 Seiten mit 79 Abbildungen und 192 Tabellen.
Geb. DM 248,–. SFr 246,–. öS 1934,40. ISBN 3-7985-0915-8.

Die ärztliche Begutachtung liegt innerhalb von 10 Jahren in 4., völlig neu bearbeiteter Auflage vor. Als das interdisziplinäre Standardwerk für den Arzt als Gutachter, Sachverständiger und Berater der sozialrechtlichen Institutionen, Gerichte und Versicherungen bietet sie das geltende rechtliche und medizinische Wissen.

Der Herausgeber und 44 kompetente Autoren haben für diese Neuauflage des Buches sämtliche Beiträge auf den neuesten Stand gebracht. Dabei wurde auch die Beziehung zu der Rechtslage in den neuen Bundesländern hergestellt. Zahlreiche aktuelle Themen wurden neu aufgenommen.

Die grundsätzliche Einteilung des Buches in sozialversicherungsrechtliche Grundlagen, privates Versicherungsrecht, pathophysiologische Grundlagen der Begutachtung und die Besonderheiten der medizinischen Fachgebiete wurde beibehalten. Ein detailliertes Sachwortverzeichnis erleichtert den Zugang zu allen Fragestellungen.

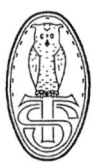

Erhältlich bei Ihrem Buchhändler.

Steinkopff Dr. Dietrich Steinkopff Verlag
Postfach 11 14 42, 64229 Darmstadt

N. **Rietbrock**, H. **Staib**, D. **Loew** (Hrsg.)

Klinische Pharmakologie

Ein Leitfaden für die Praxis

1991. 510 Seiten. 72 Abb. 139 Tab.
Geb. DM 74,–. SFr 81,50. öS 577,20.

Der Wissensstoff dieses Buches ist nach therapeutischer Systematik gegliedert und durch ein einheitliches Aufbauprinzip der Kapitel gut überschaubar. Einleitend wird das Therapieziel dargestellt, wiederkehrende Abschnitte beziehen sich auf die Eigenschaften der Arzneimittel, ihre Pharmakokinetik und Pharmakodynamik, Dosierung, unerwünschte Wirkungen und Kontraindikationen. Weitere Kapitel stellen übergeordnete Wissensinhalte dar, z. B. Arzneimittelgesetzgebung, Arzneimittelverschreibung, Arzneitherapie und Lebensalter.

„... Das Buch ist ein sehr gut gelungener, praxisbezogener Leitfaden für alle Leser, die an rationaler und sicherer Arzneimitteltherapie interessiert sind."

So urteilt die **Ärzte Zeitung**.

Erhältlich bei Ihrem Buchhändler.

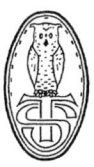

Steinkopff Dr. Dietrich Steinkopff Verlag
Postfach 11 14 42, 64229 Darmstadt

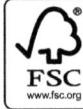

If you have any concerns about our products,
you can contact us on
ProductSafety@springernature.com

In case Publisher is established outside the EU,
the EU authorized representative is:
**Springer Nature Customer Service Center GmbH
Europaplatz 3, 69115 Heidelberg, Germany**

Printed by Libri Plureos GmbH
in Hamburg, Germany